FINAL ROUND

An Individual Health Journey with Brain Cancer

Medical conversations in this book are written as best recollected and are not direct quotes from medical personnel.

Character dialogues are reconstructed from memory and are subject to recollection capability. No intentional misrepresentation is made and specific dialogue may be inexact.

Publisher: PrintPOD Publishing

Hillsborough, New Jersey

Editor: Dina Forbes

Production Coordinator: Michael Aslett

Production Editor: Kymberly Rosenthal

Contact: printpodpub@gmail.com

Phone: 908-917-3400

Printed in the United States of America

First Edition 2019

ISBN: 978-0-578-56312-1

FINAL ROUND

An Individual Health Journey with Brain Cancer

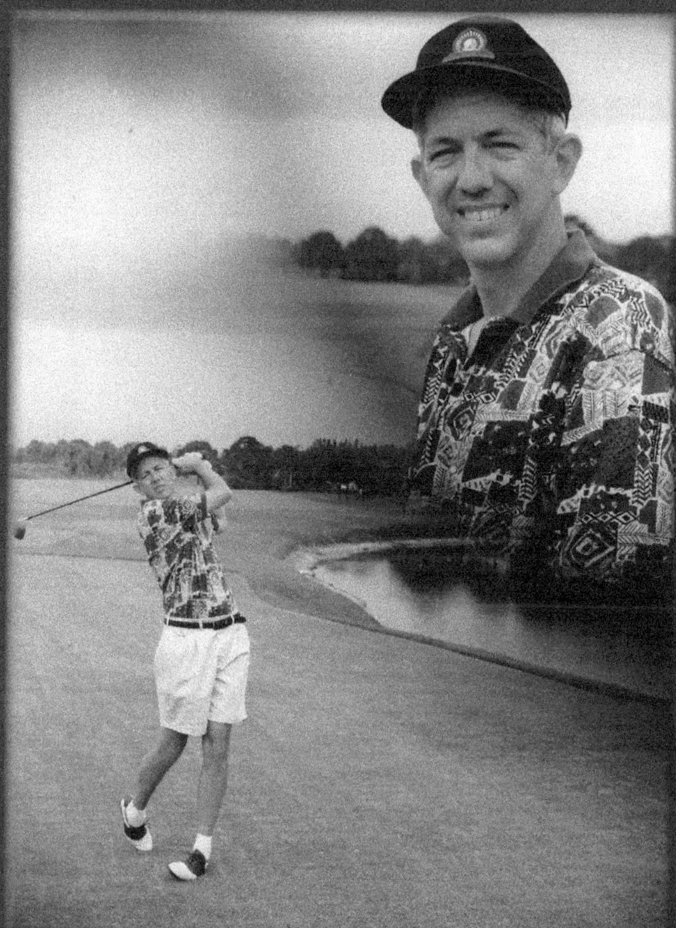

Lynn Gambill

Contents

Dedication 6

Preface 7

Chapter 1: Evaluation 9

Chapter 2: First Steps 33

Chapter 3: Getting Ready 61

Chapter 4: Follow-up 111

Chapter 5: Planning Ahead 153

Chapter 6: Setback 223

Chapter 7: Surprise 259

Chapter 8: Last Steps 313

Epilogue 329

Appendix 333

Dedication

This story is dedicated in loving memory to

Joseph Martin Gambill

June 4, 1957–January 13, 2017

In keeping with Joe's generous spirit, this story is also dedicated to the many health professionals who supported him along the way. That includes physicians, nurses, hospital staff, rehabilitation services, and hospice. May you be blessed for all you did for us and all you continue to do for others.

This is also dedicated to the many family members, friends, and neighbors who helped throughout our journey. Your caring generosity to us was overwhelming. Without you, the year would have been unbearable.

Net proceeds from the sale of this book will be donated to Massachusetts General Hospital for glioblastoma research, and to Treasure Coast Hospice.

Preface

It's said that truth is stranger than fiction. Even unintentionally distorted truth, wrung from emotions of all types, tells a story.

So, what story can be told by what Joe and I went through together throughout his journey with brain cancer? There has to be something positive that comes out of it—I refuse to believe that it was random, senseless, meaningless, or without some kind of purpose. By sharing our story, I hope to create something that may be as supportive a force in others' lives as it was a destructive one in ours.

Our situation evolved over the course of a year, followed by a complete reboot of life. We met many people, during the year and after, who had experienced gradual loss for years—sometimes decades—before the final loss. I don't know how anyone gets through it. But we seem to find the strength to do whatever is necessary to help those we love, no matter how long the illness lasts. You don't think about time when it's occurring. You only focus on how you can alleviate the pain and suffering…and provide hope, love, and caring for as long as they are with you.

My hope is that our story can show others that they're not alone—that there are many in similar circumstances and many others who will help along the way.

I also intend that this book help others in their search for information and support. Throughout Joe's illness, one of the most difficult emotions for me to cope with was the feeling of helplessness—I felt powerless to stop his pain and powerless to control what was happening to him. And not being able to easily find reliable information intensified that frustration. Between what I learned from our experience and the additional information in the appendix, I hope this book can provide tools that can help others find the resources they need to take an active role in their loved one's care. After all, knowledge is power.

Please understand that this is not written by a doctor or a professional writer. I wrote it based on the information I had access to at the time, so some of the more technical content might seem unclear, incomplete, or even inaccurate. In most cases, that information is addressed in the appendix.

If a loved one of yours is battling cancer or some other chronic, devastating illness, may you be strong, as you may have a challenging road ahead. For me, my husband's journey with brain cancer was the most difficult thing I've ever had to experience.

Chapter 1: Evaluation

Hope, whose whisper would have given
Balm to all my frenzied pain,
Stretched her wings, and soared to heaven,
Went, and ne'er returned again!

Emily Brontë

It's Tuesday, January 12, 2016. My cell phone rings at around 8:30 p.m. I'm home, half watching television, processing all that happened during the day. It's lightly snowing outside, and I'm expecting Joe to be home at around 9:30. He had an offsite meeting for work during the day, followed by a group event. So when the phone rings, I'm assuming it'll be from work or someone else in my family.

It's neither. It's Jean, a colleague of Joe's.

"Hi, Lynn," she says. "I hope you don't mind my calling you about Joe, but he doesn't seem to be himself tonight. He's having trouble standing up from his chair, and I think someone should drive him home. I hope you don't think I'm overstepping, but I'm worried about him driving home."

I ask Jean if Joe's been drinking and might be a little bit drunk, to which she replies, "I don't know exactly how much he's had, but he's behaving a little strangely, like he's a little dazed."

"It doesn't sound like he should drive," I say. "What do you suggest?"

Jean tells me their boss, Chris, drives past our house on his way home, so he and I make plans for when and where to meet. Meanwhile, their colleague Mike is going to drive Joe's car to our office and leave it in the parking lot.

I pick Joe up in the snow and ice at I-84 exit 64 in the parking lot of a Home Goods store. Joe has trouble getting out of Chris's car, and I have trouble trying to balance him so he doesn't slip on the ice. Once the car transfer is made, I drive carefully home. By this time, the snow is coming down heavily and the roads are very slippery. Fortunately, we have only a ten-minute drive to get home. I'm quizzing Joe all the way home, trying to figure out what may have happened. He tells me he may have forgotten to eat during the day, then had a couple of beers. He's so embarrassed that his boss had driven him to meet me, but he agrees that it was the best thing to do. In our garage at home, Joe has a lot of trouble standing up from the car and climbing the two steps inside. I help him with something to eat, and then we watch a little TV before we go to bed. He tells me he has a piercing headache, which makes me even more concerned—he never gets headaches, and he never expresses pain unless he's really hurting. I give him an over-the-counter medicine for the pain, and he sleeps through the night. I hope with all my heart that he's okay in the morning.

◆

By the next morning, the snow has stopped, and it's so beautiful to see the snow-coated lawn surrounding our house and the tree branches drooping under the snow load. I'm up early, and I wait to see how Joe is. He wakes up and comes out as if nothing were wrong. We start our usual morning routine, showering and getting ready for work. But I don't think Joe should go to work until he sees a doctor. I convince him to stay home, and I leave for work. Once the doctor's office is open, I call for an immediate appointment. Now, we have been patients of Dr. W—everyone in our family—for many years. We've never called with any kind of emergency or tried to see a doctor the same day we call. But when I request an appointment, I'm told to take Joe to the emergency room if we want to see a doctor today. I'm so surprised, and immediately angry. I'd been to the emergency room a few months earlier and had waited five hours until my appendix burst while I was waiting to see a doctor. *No way* am I going to let Joe be treated that way. I exchange angry words with the nurse and am very "assertive" with her. Finally, I get my way and get an appointment for Joe at noon. I pick him up from home and we go to see the doctor.

The doctor examines Joe, who of course downplays what happened. Joe leaves out that he had a "piercing" headache and hiccups and that he's having trouble standing up from a chair. He also omits that he's been more tired than usual and has been going to bed at around 9 p.m. for the last three months or so. I ask Joe about those symptoms, and he then admits to the doctor that he also has those symptoms. What is it about some men and doctors? I'm so glad I'm in the examining room with him. The doctor starts looking worried and orders an immediate MRI,* which can be done in the same building we're in. A couple of hours later, we're back in the examining room to hear the results.

The doctor is very quiet. He tells us it appears that Joe has a brain anomaly* on the right side when viewed from the rear. He schedules an urgent appointment for 4 p.m. with a neurology specialist,* Dr. K, who practices at Hartford Hospital in Connecticut. Joe and I are immediately very concerned, but we know we don't have enough information to help us understand the issue. As engineers, we want to get as much information as possible to determine what it means.

It's snowing and icing again, so the weather station is advising residents to get home before dark to avoid another incoming storm. I drive from Wethersfield to Dr. K's Farmington office in steady snow;

fortunately, there are no delays on the interstate. Joe and I are quiet as I drive. We both hold our fears inside, the worry about the storm suddenly of less consequence.

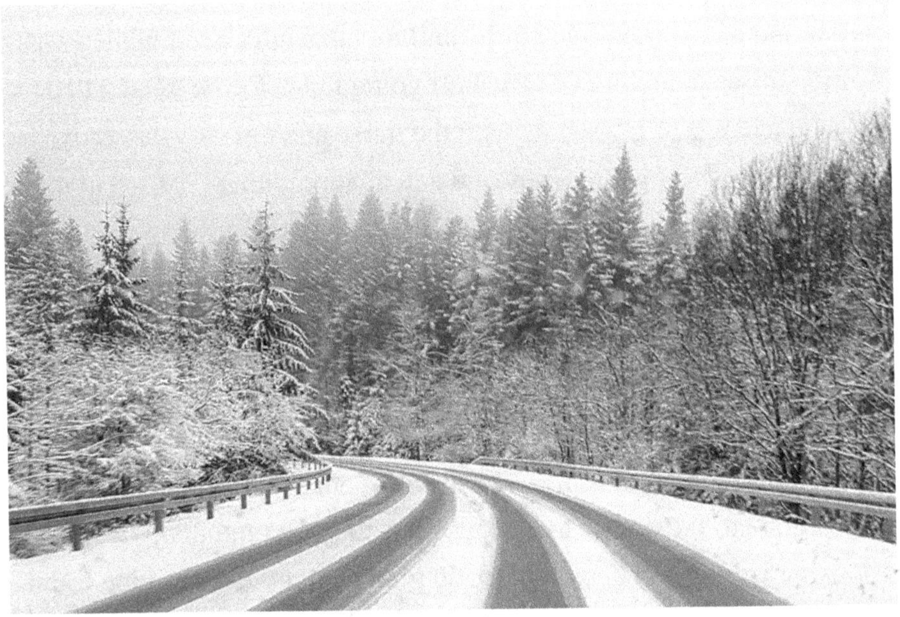

There's no one in the waiting room when we arrive. We're ushered in rather quickly and wait in the corridor outside the doctor's office. Apparently, the doctor is reviewing the results of the MRI. We wait 20 minutes or so, sitting next to each other and holding hands, until we're called into Dr. K's office. After introductions, he gets to the test results quickly. He confirms that Joe has a brain tumor,* although the exact type isn't clear from the MRI. The tumor is quite large, the size of a golf ball. Because of the location, it's consistent with Joe's symptoms: tiredness early in the evening, weakness in the legs, and headache. Dr. K recommends immediate surgery to remove the tumor; then a biopsy* of the tumor will be performed to determine what type of tumor it is. He says he believes it might be something called a *glioma** but that he can't be sure without results from the biopsy.

Dr. K is prepared to perform the surgery on Monday, January 18—Martin Luther King Jr. Day. We're stunned beyond belief at this point. Brain surgery in five days? He can tell we're shocked, but because it's snowing and almost 5 p.m., he suggests we call him in the morning for more discussion. Joe is fully functioning during all the tests and doctor's discussions. He understands all that we've been told, and we discuss what we've learned at great length on the drive home and throughout the evening. At this point, we're seriously considering having the surgery on Monday, understanding that it's important to remove the tumor as soon as possible.

In bed that night, I'm pressed close to Joe, my arm resting over his side. He's sleeping, as he's quite exhausted from the day. I can't stop thinking about what the doctors told us. I'm not sure about having such a major operation based on the findings of a neurologist we have no experience with. It's not too late, so I get back up and call my sister Peggy. A year or so ago, her husband Mike was diagnosed with throat cancer. She did some research and determined the best place for his treatment was Johns Hopkins Hospital in Baltimore. I'm wondering if we ought to go there as well.

Peggy is a huge help to me. She tells me she'll check into Joe's diagnosis and see what she can find out about specialists and which hospitals they work in. She's also going to contact a couple of her friends in the medical field and will call me in the morning with anything she finds out. I feel a lot better knowing we can get more information before we make a decision.

I also spend some time searching online to find out exactly what a glioma is. I'm dismayed by what I find: it's a type of cancer that there's no cure for. Life expectancy varies from six months to five years, but the average is around eighteen months. I find little information about how the condition progresses, but some information indicates that the usual treatment would be surgery followed by chemotherapy* and radiation.* Finding out that there's no cure and that life expectancy is so short crushes me immediately, as I never imagined Joe and I would be separated until we reached our 80s. Joe is my rock, my stability, my life's love, and my best friend. Before I completely panic, I need more information from a specialist. Maybe this isn't what I read online, I think to myself. Maybe we'll be laughing about this in a few days when we get another diagnosis. Or maybe it'll all just go away….

◆

I'm working for a man I'll call "S." He's everything you would think a career manufacturing man might be—the gruff, unyielding, direct, "get the job done yesterday and don't whine to me" type. He's also intelligent, political, and dogged. Without words, we've agreed on a work arrangement that allows both of us to function and do the job we need to do. We're both executives at an aerospace company, but he has many more years' experience in manufacturing, while 95 percent of my experience is in engineering. In theory, we should be a good team. In reality, we have worked out a division of responsibilities that best utilizes our skill sets. Sometimes, our working relationship is a little strained, although I very much respect his skills. However, I am not looking forward to a discussion with S about what is going on.

So, I don't want to talk to S. But I know I have to, because I'm going to take leave to help Joe. In the meantime, Peggy calls me to tell me that currently, several of the most well known facilities for brain tumors are at hospitals in California, Texas, and Massachusetts. One of these is at Massachusetts General Hospital in Boston, near where our son Greg works and lives. So, MGH seems like the logical choice to get a second opinion.

I research the doctors at MGH online and call for an appointment. It's around 11 a.m. on Thursday, and I'm amazed that they'll see us almost immediately—at 9 a.m. tomorrow. What great luck! Dr. N will see us—I can't believe it! I feel so much better knowing we're going to a highly renowned hospital in the country to get a second opinion.

I call Greg to explain what we know, and I spend time talking to him about Joe. I ask if we can stay with him overnight so we can drive to Boston today instead of in the morning. We both have so many questions that we hope will get answered tomorrow. I don't have enough information—just so many fears that I don't want to pass on to Greg. I want to protect my son if I can. He recently graduated from law school and has been at his first job in Boston for about a year.

I still haven't reached out to S yet, so I call and make an appointment to see him. Fortunately, I can see him in the early afternoon. I drive to work, about 20 minutes away. At this point, you may be wondering what Joe's been doing. Well, we haven't been given any particular restrictions for him. I'm concerned about his driving based on what happened Tuesday night, so I've badgered him into not driving. He seems fine around the house, although he's very concerned. He's been busy researching what he can find out about his initial diagnosis. He's quiet, and we've discussed some of his findings. He knows this is very serious. He's okay around the house, and nothing seems amiss, so I drive to work.

I arrive at S's office after parking in the main administration lot and using the back stairs. I don't want to see anyone else, because I'm not sure I can hold it together with any casual banter or work issue discussions if I run into anyone. I know what to expect from S and know this meeting will be short. Of course I have to wait once I arrive, but at least it gives me a little more time to put my game face on. Once I'm ushered into S's office, I wait while he finishes something on his computer—it's his way of showing me who's boss.

"What's up, Lynn?" he asks after joining me at his conference table.

"You may have met my husband Joe. He works in engineering," I start lamely.

"Oh yeah, I know Joe," S replies. "Isn't he in externals design?"

I reply, "Yes, he is. I took him to the doctor yesterday, and he was diagnosed with a type of brain tumor called a *glioma.*"

I tell about Joe's surgery that's scheduled for Monday and about the plans to take him to MGH for a second opinion. I explain that I'll be taking a couple of days off while Joe and I sort things out and that I'll let him know if Joe has surgery on Monday and I'll need to take more time off.

Now S is studying me closely.

"You know my wife is a nurse," he tells me. "At one time, she worked for a neurologist. I have some understanding of what you're telling me. My brother-in-law had a glioma. It was tough to treat and pretty tough on the family."

"Well, we're getting a second opinion at a well-known neurology center tomorrow and will know more then," I say. "But I plan to be with Joe for whatever he needs. I've read a little about it, so I know that a glioma can't be cured and that his time may be limited—but limited to what exactly, I don't know."

I tell S I'll be taking some time off, effective immediately. I assure him that I'll put backups in place and send him my contact information.

"Well, that should work," he replies. "Let me know when you know more."

I ask that he not discuss the situation with anyone else at work—it's very private to Joe, and he doesn't want many people to know the details of his condition. This ends the conversation, which was somewhat of a by-the-book discussion. I appreciate that S was so understanding and empathetic of the circumstances and didn't pressure me about work. I'm very relieved to be finished with the conversation. I had no big breakdown, tears gushing and all, even though I can hardly control myself. If this diagnosis is confirmed, I know I'm going to lose Joe. It's only a question of when.

My mind continues to struggle to grasp what's happening. It's so surreal. I drive home, incredibly tense, thinking about what needs to be done: pack, get gas in the car, help Joe while we travel, drive to Boston. Dinner and breakfast in Boston? How will we get to the hospital? Where will we park the car once we're there? Where is the doctor's office? *So* many things to do. I get home at around 3 p.m. and pull things together.

If I didn't know what had happened on Tuesday night and didn't know about Joe's initial diagnosis, I wouldn't know how ill he is just by looking at him. He's having trouble getting out of chairs and off the couch. He doesn't have a headache and isn't acting strangely. We'd both noticed the weakness in his legs a couple of months ago. Joe had decided it was time to start going back to the gym to see if it would help. We'd noticed this weakness in November, when we went to see Greg in Boston for Thanksgiving. We'd stayed in a bed and breakfast that had a parking lot on a steep incline. Joe's car door opened in the downward sloping direction, and he kept having trouble getting out of his Acura TLX. But other than that and starting to go to bed earlier in the evening, there were no signs at home. The weakness continued but didn't worsen. Stairs, walking, balance—all seemed fine.

Anyway, I drive us to Boston. Now, this drive is one that I've long hated. You take I-84E to I-90E and into Boston. I-84E isn't bad, but I-90E to me is a madhouse of reckless drivers and crazed semi-trucks all over the road. Add snow and ice into the mix and it can be a stressful drive. Fortunately, it was a sunny but very cold day. Joe always talks to me when I drive to Boston to help reduce my tension, chattering along the way about work, music, and books, and always with his jokes about my driving worries. This is one of the many things that make Joe the person he is. He jokes about whatever is your concern, making it seem so trivial—things like, "Look out for that red semi ahead—the driver is looking at you instead of at the road," or "Watch out over here," as he punches the inside of the passenger door.

Well, we arrive uneventfully at Greg's apartment in Brookline. Greg's roommate, Chris, is traveling, so Joe and I can use his room for the night. To access the apartment building, you go up a sloped, somewhat uneven incline. Joe navigates this pretty well, and we call Greg from the lobby to let us in remotely from his workplace. After we get through the lobby, we can use our key to get into Greg's apartment with no trouble.

Once we're inside and settled, we wait for Greg to come home from work. Joe starts messing around with the TV, and he finds a show to watch. I go into the bedroom and call his brother Jim to tell him about Joe's illness.

Joe is the oldest of three, and Jim is the youngest. There's a six-year age difference between them. Joe is close to 6'3" and weighs about 185 lbs., while Jim is about 6'4" and weighs a little over 200 lbs. Joe has a leaner build and was mostly gray by 35. Jim has a bigger build and has slightly graying hair. The family folklore is that there's some American Indian blood from several generations ago. They both have very dark eyes—almost black; are southern gentlemen; and have a dry, observant sense of humor. Hilarious to be around....

Jim is easy to talk to, and I explain the situation to him. He immediately asks how he can help. He wants to be with Joe to help in any way he can, and he asks to come to see us over the weekend. Jim and his wife live in Ashburn, Virginia, and they can drive to Connecticut in six hours or so. With the long holiday weekend coming up for Martin Luther King Jr. Day, they can get to our house Saturday and stay until Monday. We make the arrangements, and I'm so relieved to have Jim and his wife Allison come for the weekend. They're family, and I know they'll help without adding any burden to an already stressful situation.

I also call Joe's younger sister, Jane, and talk with her about Joe's diagnosis. I answer her questions as best as I can based on what we know. We discuss the best time for her to visit and agree that it will be after Joe's surgery, and I tell her we'll keep her updated whenever we find out more.

I return to the living room and sit with Joe while he watches a show, and we wait for Greg to come home. Once he joins us, we all bundle up and walk to a nearby restaurant. It's not too windy even though the temperature is close to freezing. We have a good dinner and talk about anything but the next day. I have a sinking feeling in my gut, though, as I continually think about little things that are starting to make more sense now. For example, Joe made our Christmas travel plans, and for the first time ever, he forgot to make return flights until we arrived in Florida.

◆

On Friday morning, I wake up to overcast skies and temperatures in the lower 30s in Brookline. Joe is sleeping next to me, rather soundly. We need to be at Massachusetts General Hospital for our appointment at 9 a.m. Once he's awake, Joe continues to be tired and has difficulty standing from the bed, but he can manage otherwise. We're somber, but hopeful. After a quick breakfast, I load up the car, since we'll be driving to Connecticut after the appointment. Greg is going to work today, but we'll fill him in on what the doctors tell us and plan accordingly.

I'm using my car navigation system to direct us to the hospital. Although MGH is only about four miles away, the drive takes about 30 minutes. We take Beacon Street to Storrow Drive to 55 Fruit Street—pronounced *Fruuuut* by the navigation system voice. We laugh and mimic the pronunciation. After turning on to Fruit Street, I don't know where to go. No obvious parking, no clear signs about general admittance. This is the main campus, which has nearly 30 buildings including the main hospital facility, the Lunder Building, the Yawkey Center, and the Wang Center. To say it's overwhelming would be an understatement.

I park in a parking garage, and we find an elevator to the ground floor. We walk toward what we think is the main hospital entrance. Joe has difficulty getting out of the car, but once he's standing, he can walk without issue. Throughout the walk, I'm chattering and anxious about getting to the appointment, but Joe is mostly quiet. The entrance area is crowded, and we wait our turn in line at the reception desk. We are given quick directions to our appointment in the Yawkey Building: left through the lobby, first set of elevators on the right to the 2nd floor, walk from the main hospital to Yawkey, then to another set of elevators to the 9th floor. There's a very brisk walking flow of people as we move from one building to another—many hospital staff, patients, relatives, and friends trying to maneuver around the hospital. We step out of the elevators to Dr. N's office. The waiting room is full and there's a long line to check in, but we find a couple of seats and begin to wait.

We're called into the doctor's office and are asked to wait in one of the examination rooms. I brought the CD of the MRI that was taken on Wednesday, plus Dr. K's recommendation report. We meet with a physician assistant. Now, Joe is a what you would call a "people person." As soon as the PA arrives, he perks up and is chatting with her about the weather, asking her how she's doing, and joking about my driving to MGH. She gives him a quick look at first, then relaxes and laughs at his description of my struggles to get to the hospital. She looks at his eyes and has him follow her finger left to right, up and down. She asks him to stand up, and of course he gives his very best effort and hardly has trouble standing—he wants an A+ on the exam, I suppose. She has him close his eyes, reach out with his left hand to touch his nose, and then do the same with his right hand. No comments for us. Finally, she asks him to balance on each foot. She loads the MRI into the hospital's record system and tells us the doctor will be with us shortly. We see the doctor at around 9:30 a.m.—not too bad, considering we had a 9 a.m. appointment.

First impressions are hard to go with. The doctor looks younger than I expected. He's somewhat reserved, and he seems to study us as much as we're studying him. After introductions all around, he asks about the symptoms leading up to the MRI he had reviewed. Joe describes a few things and I fill in the rest. Again, what is it about some men, not wanting to fully describe their symptoms to their doctors? Joe and I share a bit about our backgrounds and tell Dr. N that we're both engineers. Dr. N tries to make us as comfortable as he can by describing a little of his background to us—talking about data and about using tests to assess conditions. He tells us he was originally from California and has studied at Yale and Harvard, and that both of his parents were doctors in California. All the while, he's watching us as he talks to us. Finally he gets to it.

Dr. N confirms that Joe has a large mass in the frontal lobe, on the right side when looking from the rear. He uses a plastic schematic of a brain to show us where the mass is located and says it's about the size of a golf ball in diameter. The position of the mass is consistent with Joe's symptoms. Dr. N recommends that the mass be resected*

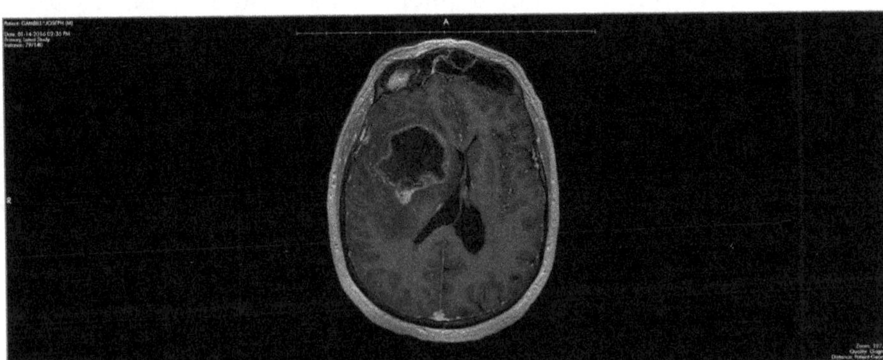

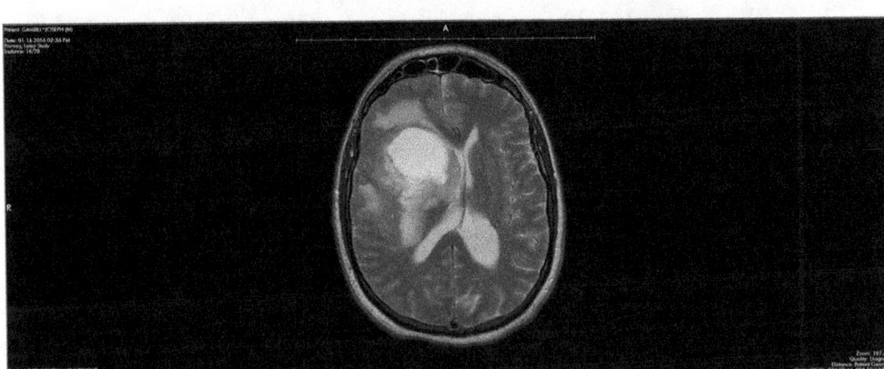

(removed) and a biopsy conducted to determine a more precise classification of the mass. He thinks Joe should start taking steroids* to reduce the size of the mass and anti-seizure medicine in preparation for the surgery. If Joe has any pain, the doctor tells us, he should continue taking over-the-counter pain medicine but no non-steroidal anti-inflammatory drugs (NSAIDs) like aspirin, ibuprofen, or naproxen.

Dr. N says that since many of his colleagues will be on holiday for Martin Luther King Jr. Day on Monday, he'd like to schedule the surgery for Tuesday so he can have his best team members working with him. He knows we've consulted with a neurosurgeon* in Hartford, but he doesn't push us to come to MGH. He does tell us about the capabilities available at MGH, for both surgery and follow-up care. He explains that chemotherapy and radiation treatment will likely follow but that the extent and exact nature will be determined based on the surgery and biopsy results. He also tells us that, based on his experience, the mass is likely a type of tumor called a *glioblastoma**. We don't know exactly what a glioblastoma is, but we've read a little about it based on the initial diagnosis. We know the condition and the surgery are very serious.

Dr. N explains that the surgery is likely going to take four to five hours and that they'll use a real-time MRI to guide the resection. We ask what will happen if we do nothing, and the doctor explains that Joe will have a limited time if we decide not to treat him. He tells us he can't say exactly how much time but that he believes the surgery and subsequent treatment will provide the best chance for Joe to have a longer life. How much longer depends on so many factors, and each case is different, he says. We try to get him to be more specific, but he says he won't go down that path with us. It's absolutely not what we want to hear, and Joe and I are both devastated. We have to decide if we want treatment in Boston or Hartford. We know we don't have time to even think everything over, never mind talk about it, so we ask if we can get back to him in a few hours. He gives us a direct phone number to reach him, and we thank him before we go to the waiting room.

Joe and I are practical people. We're educated, and we work as professionals in the aerospace industry. We understand what we've been told, and we're aware of the surgery risks. But we don't understand how much the surgery may help in the long term, and we're concerned about Joe's quality of life post surgery and with the follow-up treatment. Joe understands all of this—his thought processes are not compromised. Ultimately, it'll be his decision. We talk over all the choices, including not having surgery. Joe thinks not having surgery isn't truly an option, and I agree. As serious as the surgery is, we both believe it's the best option. The next step is to decide where to have the surgery. So Joe says it in the best way.

"We can have the surgery in Hartford, and it'll be more convenient logistically," he says. "Or we can return to MGH and come to a well known hospital for brain cancer treatment. We'd be just plain lazy to opt for Hartford."

Now, I understand about the logistics of having medical issues addressed in Boston. Our son Greg had six surgeries in Boston to correct a sleep apnea issue. It was pure hell, and traveling into and out of Boston regularly for a year and a half was a nightmare. I agree with Joe, but I know it's going to be incredibly difficult. It takes us a couple of hours to talk it all through; then we contact Dr. N to ask him to help us. He agrees, and we commit to surgery at MGH on Tuesday, January 19, 2016.

But our day is not over—far from it. Fortunately, the doctor's office helps us with the insurance approvals. But we still need to notify Greg, Joe's family, Joe's boss, my boss, my family, and our friends. So we leave Boston at around 3 p.m. and get home to Connecticut a couple of hours later. The drive is exhausting, and there's excessive traffic leaving Boston for the long weekend. Joe rests for a bit on the way home while I fret about the drive. We're supposed to be back in Boston in time for Joe to have another MRI done on Monday. There are so many things to address before we leave—having prescriptions filled, packing for the hospital, getting food for the weekend, finding someone who'll take care of our pets while we're away… I'm also answering work phone calls and directing them to other people as issues come up.

I'm so upset, and all I can think about is how to make it all go away so Joe will be okay. The thought of losing him is unfathomable. Joe is everything to me—my love, my best friend, my sounding board, my only refuge in a life (of my choosing) that is complex and taxing. I love him more than anything in this world (except our son, which is a different kind of love.) In three short days, our world has been completely rocked and turned upside down. It's as if I'm looking at someone else's life—as if I'll wake up and everything will be sane again. I realize that although Joe is capable of making decisions, he's also overwhelmed. What can he do but hope that everything will return to normal? He's already talking about going back to work after the surgery. He wants so badly to have things be as they were.

When I call Joe's brother Jim, he firms up plans to see us for the weekend. Greg is going to come home from Boston on Saturday to spend time with us and to help me take Joe to Boston Monday.

After dinner, Joe and I continue to look up everything we can find out about glioblastoma online. At the time, we weren't aware of how to find accurate, reliable medical information online, so we rely on Wikipedia.* I'm not comprehending everything that I read, but I understand enough to know it's a type of brain cancer that can be treated in some circumstances, although it's incurable. Glioblastoma, according to Wikipedia, is the *most aggressive cancer* that begins within the brain. *The average length of survival is twelve to fifteen months*, with fewer than three percent to five percent of people surviving longer than five years. *Without treatment, survival is typically three months.* There's a lot more in Wikipedia, but I'm focused on those statements. Joe is reading it also, and he truly looks dazed as he researches more and more. Neither of us realized all this based on any of our doctor's discussions. But now I think I understand why we were scheduled to see a neurosurgeon at MGH so quickly and why surgery was scheduled for Tuesday.

Nothing seems important at this point except how to help Joe. How do we find a path for him to beat those odds? I understand that the life that we knew up until this point is on hold, maybe even over. Joe has hopes he'll return to what he loves to do. I also know there are so many things that have to be prepared for, the most important being Joe's needs and comfort.

We go to bed together and hold each other close. We're both crying and telling each other how much we love each other. Joe doesn't seem as sick as the diagnosis suggests. His symptoms just aren't that dramatic. Could the diagnosis still be a mistake?

◆

I usually wake up earlier than Joe. Saturday morning is no exception, and I'm groggy and slow moving. I start thinking about what I'll do today, thinking about going out to work. It's been my routine for so long, and I start to think about getting ready to go. Then, something like a gray mist encompasses me and I remember that everything has changed in our lives. My chest tightens, and my breath is shorter. My husband has terminal brain cancer, with a finite time to live. Things like this don't happen to people like us. We're both well respected in our fields, with 37 years of experience each in the aerospace industry. We're both in managerial positions at work. We're used to helping others with their personal situations, not *having* personal problems ourselves. And if we do, we take them in stride. But this is different. I know there's only one way it can end, and it's a question of how long we have.

I prepare myself for the day. How will Joe feel today? I think about breakfast, getting a few things ready for Jim and Allison, Greg's arrival today…and more research on Joe's diagnosis.

Joe gets up, showers, dresses, and walks into the kitchen. He gets himself a diet soda. This is what he starts every day with. He gets his cereal and sits at the table with me. He's fully functioning…he reads the paper, and we comment on this and that. He takes the new medicines that were prescribed, along with his medicines for Crohn's disease,* high blood pressure, and high cholesterol. He's now taking five medicines, all on different schedules. This would be hard for anyone to keep up with. So I go upstairs and make a computer spreadsheet, listing the times to take each medicine every day. I create boxes to check off so he can keep up with what he needs to do. I bring it downstairs to him and he scoffs at it, saying, "I can remember this!" But I know I need to make sure it's done correctly, and this is the only way I can keep it straight.

Now, Joe and I spend a lot of time working. Greg is our only son, and he's finished with his various academic achievements and is working full time. He started college in 2007, so he's spent less and less time living with us over the years. It was a tough adjustment when he went to college. We both missed him so much, and we found that we began spending more time together and more time at work. Our plan had been to retire when I was 62, which is three years away. We live somewhat austerely for what we earn. We save a lot, but we haven't really put together a more formal retirement plan. We always told each other we would, but with our priorities often being our jobs, we never got around to it. We also never finished our estate planning, which we had started in 2009. And Joe had a few loose ends to close as executor of his parents' wills—he'd lost his mother and father in 2006 and 2007, respectively. Now we're faced with the most major of medical issues and we don't have our act together. We both know it, and we talk about what we need to do. I have so many fears about the upcoming surgery, and I don't know what Joe's capability will be after the surgery. But I keep these thoughts to myself. After all, it's a major brain surgery—will he be the same as he was before? I don't know. We outline the steps we need to take. It really helps us to focus our minds on something so that we don't dwell over what's coming on Tuesday.

We also talk about the possibility of a negative outcome from the surgery. Joe tells me very clearly that he really wants to return to work *if possible*. He also tells me he wants to keep the specific nature of his illness private, as he doesn't want to be treated differently when he returns to work or by those he knows. But he doesn't want to spend his remaining time in Connecticut—he wants to return to Florida, where we lived for many years before moving to Connecticut with our company. We already have a home in Florida. But in December, we decided to put it on the market, and now we have a contract with a new home in an area a little farther north. We're closing on the new home next month. We talk about canceling the new home contract, but then we decide it's where we want to spend our remaining time together. Our current Florida home isn't well suited to daily living, and the other is a much better layout. It also has many amenities, such as golf, which Joe wants to try to do more of after we move if his health permits. So we've discussed the major extraneous issues we need to systematically address and decided on what we'll do.

◆

Jim and Allison arrive close to 5 p.m. on Saturday. The drive took longer than expected, but at least they're here now. It's such a help to have them here. Joe and Jim really get along and enjoy each other. Allison brought a dinner from a meal delivery service, and we decide to have it tomorrow night. Tonight, at Joe's request, we're going to his favorite restaurant in Ellington, Trattoria Da Lepri. Greg arrives at around 6 p.m., and we leave for the restaurant. Joe is okay, but I can tell he's tired. He has a lot of difficulty getting up from his chair to go to the car. He has no problem going down the two steps to get to the car in the garage, but when we park at the restaurant, he really has to work at standing up from the car. Jim, ever thoughtful, sees this and helps his brother. We've been regulars at this restaurant over the past year and a half, and the owner's father greets us as we come in. We exchange pleasantries and complain about the cold weather before being seated at a nice table in the second room, with Joe next to me and Jim, Allison, and Greg across the table.

Both Joe and Jim are graduates of the University of Tennessee. Joe attended the Outback Bowl in Tampa on New Year's Day earlier in the month, and he describes the game to Jim. UT won by a score of 45-6, finishing the season with a 9-4 record. He met a couple of his longtime friends, Bennett and John, at the game and they did their usual overzealous fan routine, yelling until they were hoarse at the various plays during the game. I suspect there was a fair amount of drinking during the game as well. Jim tells us about his recent travels with his job, and Allison and Jim talk about the transition they've been making coming back to work in the U.S. after being expats in Singapore for seven years. Greg is a vegan and talks to us about his food choices these days, and I try not to be his mother and voice concerns about getting enough calories and protein in his diet. I know if I condemn his diet it will only push him more toward it. There's an undercurrent at dinner, but we all ignore it and act as if everything is perfectly normal. Joe has been getting headaches in the evening when he seems more tired.

The rest of the weekend goes well. A couple of times, Jim and Allison individually ask me what they can do to help, and they offer any support I ask for. None of us know what to plan for, so it's a standing offer. We don't know how long Joe will be in the hospital, as it depends on how the surgery goes. Talking with Jim and Allison about what the doctors have told us is very helpful to me. They're both well-educated professionals working as consultants for project evaluation using their chemical engineering backgrounds. They're practical, grounded, and sensible. It's a relief to discuss what we know at this point.

◆

It's Sunday, January 17, and I'm relieved that Greg, Jim, and Allison are here with us. I know I can leave Joe and that he's in good hands while I'm gone, so I get up earlier than everyone else and slip out to attend Mass. I'm Catholic, and my faith was really tested when my son Greg had to have surgery to correct his sleep apnea. What was supposed to be one surgery ended up being six for various reasons, the biggest being bone infection after the jaw surgeries. I can't remember how many times I prayed various versions of novenas to St. Jude. And I'm forever thankful for these prayers being answered.

Now I'm in church praying for Joe's health to be restored. I can't understand how Joe, of all people, could have such a severe illness. He's the best person I know, and I can't believe he's going through this. I pray for his surgery to be successful and for this awful disease to be overcome.

Joe and Jim spend time during the day exchanging various childhood stories. One in particular that they often tell is about Joe's visit to their Aunt Patricia's house and staying with their cousin Jimbo. One night when they're about 12 years old, they pretend to be asleep when Aunt Patricia checks on them. As soon as they're sure she's convinced that they're asleep, they climb out a window in Jimbo's room so they can go to the closest main road and shoot off firecrackers to scare drivers. One thing leads to another, with an irate driver chasing them through the woods as they scramble back to the house and climb back into the window. As Jimbo reaches his hand through the window, he feels something on the other side and snatches his hand away. He whispers to Joe that he thinks someone is in his bed—and that it may be his mother. What to do? They consider their choices and realize they've been caught. There's nothing they can do except climb into the window and own it. An inquisition by Jimbo's mother is followed by many denials of any wrongdoing—except, of course, leaving the house. A story Joe and Jimbo told at many family get-togethers over the years....

Joe and Jim also chat about their childhood and their parents, Ed and Sarah. It's so great that Jim can be here with Joe. Joe talks to Jim about things in our house that belonged to their parents, and he offers his brother anything he wants.

Greg and I drive to my office to pick up Joe's car, which was left in the parking lot Tuesday night when Joe's boss drove him to meet me. On the way there, Greg and I talk about the upcoming surgery. We both know that there's a chance the surgery won't be successful, and it's devastating to know we could lose Joe as soon as Tuesday.

We have a family dinner on Sunday night. Allison cooks the meal from the delivery service, which we all enjoy. We're careful to talk about almost anything but the upcoming surgery. Lots of joking around. Joe, Jim, and Greg are all great imitators. They spend some time mimicking various golf friends' swings and stances, as well as one another's. They set up the practice putting game and have a competition. I don't remember who ends up with bragging rights after the game, but there's plenty of trash talking going on.

Joe retires early, at around 9 p.m., and the rest of us hold our thoughts to ourselves as we prepare to end the evening.

Chapter 2: First Steps

Do not go gentle into that good night,
Old age should burn and rave at close of day;
Rage, rage against the dying of the light.

Dylan Thomas

It's Monday, January 18, 2016—the start of Joe's medical treatment at Massachusetts General Hospital in Boston. He's supposed to check in today, with tests to be conducted in preparation for tomorrow's surgery. We're checking the weather constantly this time of year, trying to avoid snow and ice storms when we travel. The weather forecast is generally about 50 percent accurate in terms of storm severity, but if a storm is in the forecast, it usually arrives within a day or so of predictions. Today, it's supposed to snow in Boston midday.

I'm out of bed early, packing what I think we'll need. I have no idea how long we'll be in Boston after the surgery, so it's hard to know how much to bring. I plan to stay in the hospital with Joe for as long as they'll let me and I can be helpful. I know that I can go to Greg's apartment whenever I need to, and I can always wash a few things there if I don't pack enough clothes. Packing for Joe is much easier. He needs something to wear into the hospital and something to wear when we return. Because it's so cold, we'll need gloves, hats, neck scarves, coats, snow boots, sweaters, and long pants.

I pack the car, fill up the tank at the gas station, return home, and make breakfast. We're mostly ready to go once Joe and Greg are up and have breakfast. Jim and Allison plan to leave at around 9:30 a.m., with us leaving just behind them. It'll take about two hours to get to the hospital, and I want to miss the snowstorm.

Like the last couple of days, Joe wakes up and seems to feel reasonably well. He still has weakness in his legs, but three days of taking the prescribed steroids seems to be helping him. He has no loss of balance, and he isn't saying he has a headache. He continues to have hiccups, but not quite as frequently. Breakfast is a bit more somber than last night. We're all a little on edge, and I'm especially apprehensive. Between the drive to Boston, the impending snowstorm, navigating the hospital, and making sure Joe is okay all the while, I'm wound pretty tight. We have two cats that need care while we're away, and I made arrangements with Greg's friend Colin to check on them. I'm sure I'm forgetting something we need, but I've prepared as much as I can at this point. Greg and Joe are made from the same mold when it comes to traveling. They're both very low-key and take things as they come. Today is no different.

Jim and Allison load their car for their drive back to Ashburn. Greg also packs his car, as he'll be following us to Boston. I'm eager to leave so we can avoid the snow. There's a lot of running up and down stairs as everything is made ready, but Joe is sitting at the dining room table because I've forbidden him from doing anything else. "She who must be obeyed," he quips.

When Jim and Allison are ready to leave, Jim approaches Joe. "Bro, thanks for letting us drop in on you like this. I'll be thinking about you today and especially tomorrow. You take care of yourself, and I want to see you again real soon."

He makes good eye contact with Joe, which Joe returns. The two do a "man hug," and Jim pats his brother's back.

“So glad you came to see me,” Joe says. “It was a good weekend.”

These two aren’t exactly good at communicating their feelings at this point, but what they’re really telling each other is palpable, even if the words aren’t there. There’s real love between these two brothers. Joe walks Jim to the door and down the steps to Jim and Allison’s car. Joe walks to the back of the car and makes grand gestures directing Jim on how to back out of the driveway—his left arm straight out from his shoulder, right arm moving in a full circle. Their father always did the same when the boys visited their parents. Jim understands what Joe is doing, and he honks his car horn in acknowledgment as they leave.

The rest of us leave for Boston about 30 minutes later, closer to 10 a.m. I end up following Greg. He knows his way around the city much better than I do, and even with the navigation system giving me directions, it’s much easier to follow him. We stop for lunch in Brookline before we go to the hospital—last chance for Joe to have something other than hospital food for a while. We stop at Anna’s Taqueria near Greg’s apartment. It’s not too crowded, and we enjoy a couple of fresh wraps before we drive to the hospital.

When we were at the hospital on Friday, we discovered the Fruit Street Garage, which was closest to the hospital’s main entrance. Today, Greg and I easily find parking spots there. Once again, we take the elevator to the ground floor, walk across the street, and walk through the main entrance. To my surprise, the hospital entrance is much quieter than it was on Friday. We stop at the check-in desk in the main lobby, but they don’t seem to have a record of Joe being scheduled to check in today. The admitting staff seems to be the “B” team, and they’re bewildered. I insist that they call Dr. N’s office and see what’s going on. We wait for close to 45 minutes before they reach someone who knows and Joe can be admitted. The staff directs us to the Lunder Building, and we navigate to the correct area on the 6th floor. With no one to ask along the way, finding the room is harder than it had been on Friday. Finally, at almost 4 p.m., Joe is in his assigned room.

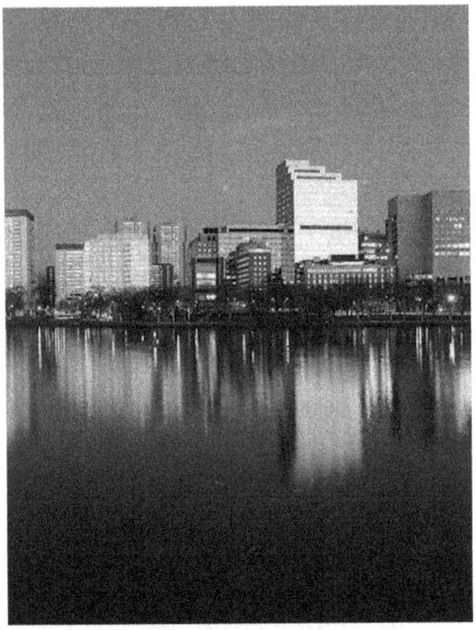

We wait in the hospital room for what seems like a long time, but it's really only an hour or so. Joe has changed into his very attractive hospital gown and nonslip blue socks. We meet one nurse, but she has no specific orders for Joe yet. Eventually we're told that Joe's scheduled MRI will be performed at 9 p.m. and that one of the doctors on weekend duty will stop by at some point to meet Joe. We were hoping to see Dr. N, but we're told that won't happen until tomorrow morning. Joe's surgery is scheduled for 7 a.m. Joe and Greg are just chilling out watching TV, and I decide to go the hospital chapel. They continue to act as if things are perfectly normal—as if they're home catching up on sports. I guess it's the best you can do when things are out of your control.

On my way to the chapel, I spot a man of the cloth. He appears to be a Catholic priest, but I may be presumptuous. He seems to be making his rounds. He sees me and asks if he can be of any assistance. I pause, as I'm not sure what Joe would think about a chaplain visiting him. Joe was brought up Methodist and attends Catholic Mass with me a couple of times a year—for the "big events" like Christmas and Easter. The chaplain introduces himself as *Father*, so I assume he's Catholic. I ask him to visit Joe, and I explain a little about the situation. He understands that Joe isn't Catholic, and I ask him if he can give Joe the sacrament of Anointing of the Sick. He agrees and says he'll stop by shortly.

Back in the room, I explain to Joe what I did. His eyes actually tear up, and he thanks me. I'm so surprised.

Some food arrives for Joe, his last meal before surgery tomorrow. It's some kind of chicken with steamed vegetables and bread. Of course Greg cracks jokes about hospital food, but Joe says it really isn't too bad. While he's finishing up, the chaplain knocks on the door. I wave him in, and he introduces himself to Joe and Greg.

I'm a little apprehensive about what the chaplain will say. But he goes with the flow a little and watches TV for a minute with Joe and Greg. He asks Joe about his upcoming surgery, and Joe explains what he knows. The chaplain then talks to Joe about being afraid.

"Fear is useless; we fear those things we don't understand and can't control," he says. "Think about the love in this room from your family, and know that they'll always be with you. Consider the positive: you're in good hands here at MGH."

He continues, "Also, trust in your faith. God is with you and will stay by your side."

He then tells Joe he's going to administer the sacrament of the sick, also known as anointing of the sick. The sacrament, he explains, provides comfort, peace, courage, and even forgiveness of sins. He conducts the sacrament, wishes us the best, and quietly leaves. Once again, Joe isn't Catholic, but he thanks me for having the chaplain see him. He says he appreciated what the chaplain said to him and that it helped him.

At a little after 9 p.m., an orderly comes to take Joe for his MRI. I ask if I can go as well, and I'm allowed.

At this point, Greg walks over to Joe's bed, hugs him, and tells him, "Dad, I'll see you tomorrow. I'll be here first thing in the morning before they take you to surgery. I love you."

Both Joe's and Greg's eyes are misting. Joe gives his son a fist bump and says, "See you tomorrow. Love you too."

The orderly takes us down completely empty hallways, through various double doors, and finally to an elevator that isn't public. It's large inside to accommodate multiple hospital beds, and it moves slowly as we go down a couple of floors. We exit and make a few more turns, finally arriving at a large area with what appears to be two rooms—one room to wait in and the other, glass enclosed, with a very large MRI machine. The area is completely empty of people except for two men in white hospital overcoats. The whole setup, including the trip to the MRI area, is kind of creepy. I've never been to a hospital area where there were no other patients. Joe's wristband is checked, computers are used to confirm the testing to be done, and the MRI technicians explain the process.

The test process will take more than an hour. The technicians ask Joe if he's claustrophobic, and he says that he is slightly. He wasn't prescribed any medicine to help him relax as we didn't know to ask for it, not realizing how long the test would take. When we ask why his first MRI took only about fifteen minutes, they tell us this MRI equipment has much greater imaging capability and provides many more snapshots of the brain. This equipment will give the surgeon the higher-fidelity baseline assessment of the surgical location and surrounding area.

The technicians tell Joe that it's really important that he not move during the testing. They say they'll talk to him during the process and let him know how it's going and will use semisoft bolsters to keep his head in place, with others under the small of his back and under his knees. They explain that if he moves, they'll have to repeat the test series. That resonates with Joe, and he's determined to get the test over with as quickly as possible.

The testing proceeds, without any repeat testing required. When it's over, Joe is very stiff from being in the same position for so long and has some welcome relief when he's transferred to his hospital bed. An orderly returns, and we travel back to Joe's room through the solitude of the hospital elevator and corridors. Joe talks to the orderly about the upcoming Super Bowl, asking him whether he's rooting for the Broncos or the Panthers. They talk about football on the way back to the room and I zone out, since I'm not very interested in the subject.

The evening concludes with lights out after I make up a sleeping space on a pullout seating area that doubles as a twin bed. There are sheets and pillows for me to use, and I'm so thankful I can stay in the hospital with Joe. Already his arm has been prepped and he's connected to fluids for the surgery tomorrow. But we don't talk about the surgery. We both know what's coming.

I tell Joe I love him and that he'll be just fine during and after the surgery. I confirm with him our decision to come to MGH for surgery and follow-up care, and he agrees. Nonetheless, I'm terrified for Joe, and I think he's afraid too, although it's not like him to express fear. My job is to reassure him that everything will be all right. The last thing he needs is to have to try to console me.

◆

The next morning, the noises of the hospital—low voices, carts rolling down corridors, the occasional clatter of who knows what—make it hard to sleep. I'm already sitting up by around 5:30 a.m., dressed for the day, not sure when someone will come by to see Joe. A group of doctors, none of whom we've met, stop in at around 6 a.m. At least one of them is on the same neurological team as Dr. N, and it appears a couple of them might be medical residency students, maybe one from the hospital staff. The introductions are fast. Joe's vital signs* were checked and we were told that the anesthesiologist* would be stopping by shortly. You do a lot of waiting in the hospital, and that's exactly what we do.

A man in his early thirties comes in to the room, greeting us with a smile and a "good morning." He introduces himself and asks Joe general questions about his health, including any allergy history or prior problems with anesthesia. He also asks Joe if he could remember what he'd been given in the past, to which Joe replied that he'd been given propofol* without issue. The doctor explained that he would be careful when he was inserting a tube into Joe's throat so he could breathe while he was unconscious from the anesthetic, to help avoid a sore throat afterward. He added that he'd use an anti-nausea medicine to prevent him from vomiting during surgery.

Greg arrives, and we're told we can accompany Joe to the pre-op waiting area. We have to take all our belongings from the room because Joe might be brought to a different room post-surgery, so we gather our belongings and are ready when an orderly arrives a few minutes later.

We go through more back corridors and elevators to get to the pre-op area, but this time there are a lot of people around. Greg and I follow the bed Joe is being pushed on through what seems to be a maze of corridors. Once we're in the pre-op area, a couple of nurses stop by, one at a time but asking the same questions: "Can you tell me your name?" "What time is it?" "Why are you here today?" And they each carefully compare his hospital wristband with their paperwork. Joe jokes with them and asks them if they're asking him trick questions. One nurse smiles, but the other doesn't. The anesthesiologist stops by again. He explains more about the anesthesia process and says the surgery will take five to six hours.

The anesthesiologist leaves, and Dr. N stops by just as Joe is being prepped for surgery. He's brief and is clearly focused on the surgery—all business, and no time for jokes or bonding. He tells me he'll call me in the waiting room after surgery to let me know how the surgery goes and reminds us that he'll be performing a right craniotomy* to resect the tumor and perform a biopsy on it. There are many disclaimer documents for Joe to sign, listing a multitude of things that could go wrong—paralysis, partial loss of motor control, speech impediment, memory impairment…the list is long and quite scary. We read the paperwork carefully, and Joe sticks with the decision to proceed. After all, we're pretty sure what will happen if nothing is done. So Joe is wheeled off to the operating room.

I'm completely panicked when Joe is gone. I try to be positive, because I don't want Greg to see how worried I am. He's only 26—too young to see a parent in such a serious situation. I know I need to be strong for him. But I'm so afraid I'll never see Joe again or that he will never be the same again after his surgery. That he'll lose parts of himself that I so love. Oh, why is this happening? Why can't it be me instead? Why Joe? He's the best person I know—why him? Why didn't I realize sooner that he was sick? Would it have made a difference? So many thoughts, so many self-incriminations… This goes through my mind quickly. But I do know that none of these thoughts will change the circumstances and that I need to focus on how to help Joe and Greg, so I try to get control of myself. Together, Greg and I wander around trying to find the waiting area. We need to be sure we're in the right place so the doctor can reach me later.

Eventually we find the waiting area in the Cox Building. It's very crowded, and there are few places left to sit. There are a few long cushioned seats with people stretched out trying to sleep. I long for some sleep, knowing I can't do anything but pray and think about Joe's surgery being a success. I brought my great-grandmother's rosary that my dad gave me when Greg was going through his dental surgeries. It has an 18k gold cross with amethyst beads, worn from years of use. I conceal the rosary in my hand in case I fall asleep. I'm not confident that something won't be stolen here, although I have no basis other than my lack of familiarity to cause this concern. Greg and I are both on edge, and he goes looking for coffee and something to eat. I close my eyes and wait.

As much as I'd like to sleep, I can't. I'm so anxious about the surgery that my mind slips from present to past, almost at random. Five hours is a long time to wait. I start thinking about the early years with Joe, before we were married.

We both worked for the same aerospace company and were hired within a few weeks of each other to work in their Florida office. The company had some new, large government contracts but didn't have sufficient staff to accommodate them. They hired close to 300 engineers, mostly recent college graduates, in about a year's time. For retention reasons, the recruits were mostly from the South, although a few were from the New England area.

Because there were so many new hires, we ended up developing activities that we could participate in. There was beach volleyball, co-ed softball, co-ed basketball, water skiing, golf, scuba diving, and running, among others. There were also many happy-hour events that typically took place on a Friday after work. Because we were all new hires, some of our college habits carried over. We worked from 7:30 a.m. to 4 p.m. each day. During daylight saving time, we had a lot of time in the afternoon to pursue other activities.

> One Friday, there's a promotion party for a colleague at the Abbey Road on Military Trail and PGA Boulevard…meaning we should meet for happy hour at Abbey Road. The word is out, and all the newbies know about it. There's about an eight percent population of women recently hired, so as usual, the word gets to us quickly. A group of us girls decide to go.
>
> The room is so packed with people that it's a challenge to walk through the crowd. The tallest in the crowd can look around and see who's here. At 6'3", Joe can see above most of the crowd. Because there are only a few women present, we're quickly noticed. We can't reach the bar to get a drink without a lot of pushing and shoving, so we're slowly making our way to the bar when Joe approaches us.
>
> "Hey girls, how are you doing?" he drawls with his southern accent. "You can't raise your arm in here without hitting someone from work. Y'all work at the plant?"

> Joe makes eye contact with each of us, grinning an easy smile. We nod our heads, confirming that we all work at the same place. He offers to get us drinks at the bar, and we accept. It's a relief to have someone fight the crowd for us.
>
> Joe delivers our drinks safely and jokes about how he didn't spill a drop. "That would be a terrible waste," he says.
>
> We compare information about our departments and our thoughts about work. We all agree it's exciting to be in West Palm Beach, living in Florida, and working on aerospace engine design. When some of Joe's friends join us, our group grows to ten or so. My friends and I leave after about an hour to meet some other friends for dinner, but I'll always remember the first time I met Joe and his relaxed, personable way of conversing.

I'm nodding off in the reception area, too keyed up to really sleep, not to mention uncomfortable. The waiting room is equipped with monitors that list the patient surgery number and a status, such as *pre-op, in surgery,* or *in recovery*. Joe is in surgery for more than five hours before the monitor indicates he's in recovery. Then I wait another half hour before my phone rings.

It's Dr. N, and he gets directly to the point: the tumor has been removed, and the surgery was a success. He says he removed 99 percent of the tumor, but only those areas that would not impact motor skills, such as speech and walking. The initial pathology* of the tumor confirmed the tumor was a glioma, but the results of an additional evaluation in a few days will provide more specific information.

I thank Dr. N profusely before I hang up, but my hands are shaking so much that I can hardly put my phone away. I'm so relieved he said the surgery was a success. I'm eager to see Joe, but even though Dr. N said I'll be able to see him in the recovery area in about 45 minutes, I know from my son's surgeries that he's very unlikely to be responsive and coherent for the rest of the day. That doesn't mean I don't want to see him as soon as I can. I want to see that he's breathing, see his skin tone, and generally check on the nurse attendance for him. I've learned that a patient whose family and friends check in regularly will get better care, and I want Joe to have the very best medical attention.

Eventually a volunteer from the main reception area calls my name and tells me I can go see Joe. She directs me to go to the 6th floor of the Lunder Building, where there's a recovery area close to the elevator exit. Navigating around the hospital is very uncomfortable, as there are now swarms of people walking at various paces. Greg and I are among the bewildered, searching our way around, while others walk to their destinations with determination. We're both so tense that we snipe at each other in our frustration trying to find our way. Turn left, long corridor to walk down, veer right again, take elevator to 2nd floor, get off long corridor, turn left, turn right to another bank of elevators to 6th floor.

We arrive at the recovery room, both with raw emotions. The entryway is locked, so I use a phone next to the door to call and am told we can see Joe in about fifteen minutes. Greg and I each take a seat in a small waiting area nearby, close to an indoor atrium. I can see through the glass that the sky is clear, although I know the outside temperature is very cold.

My phone rings—we can go see Joe now. I use the phone on the wall near the entry door again, and this time it opens for us. On the right is a semi-circular desk area lined with several computers, where various nurses are watching the screens. On the left and in front of us are hospital beds, most of which are occupied. Some of the beds are surrounded by curtains hanging from the ceiling. I approach the desk area and ask to see Joe. The nurse checks her computer to see where he is and who his attending nurse is, and she tells us someone will see us shortly.

We stand and wait. I think I spot Joe. Ahead and to my right. A nurse is checking his fluids and his vital signs, and she looks tired. I approach his bed as she looks up. Joe's head, including his ears and forehead, is completely wrapped in white gauze. His eyes are closed, and he has a breathing tube in his mouth. His skin appears pallid, but it could be the overhead lighting in the area. In his left arm, an IV is connected to multiple bags of fluids. His body is covered with several white hospital blankets, and I can see the connection from the base of the bed to the compression boots on his feet and legs. His body is supported by the bed at an incline, so his upper body is raised.

I'm outwardly calm—this is what I expected to see. After all, my son had six major dental surgeries; being in the recovery room and seeing someone you love so much unconscious is never easy, but at least this isn't the first time I've seen this. The things I fear are nausea, seizures, and convulsion, but Joe appears to be sedate. I'm not relieved at all, but I understand that what I'm seeing may be what to expect at this stage.

I tell the nurse that I'm Joe's wife, and I ask how he's doing. I'm struck again by how tired she appears. She tells me all his vital signs are as they should be and that she'll remove the breathing tube in a few hours, after observing him. He'll have a catheter* in place until sometime tomorrow, and they might be able to move him to his own room in a couple of hours. I ask her how the surgery went. She tells me that a doctor will be coming to his room late in the afternoon and we can ask any questions we have then, but that as far as she knows, things went well.

None of this is particularly consoling to me. What I'm really worried about is what will happen when Joe wakes up, and the next couple of days. The first step is the surgery, and hoping there are no complications from it. The next step is—what about Joe being Joe? My mind becomes frantic to even think that he may not be himself. That the surgery may have changed him in some way he can't recover from. I know, I know, useless and negative thinking, but I can't control my worry. It's been one week since I picked him up from the parking lot in front of the Home Goods store. So much change, so quickly….

As I look at Joe, I think about his beautiful smile, clever words, and dancing black eyes. I think about the Christmas holiday, only three weeks ago. Joe and I had put up our artificial Christmas tree a few days after Thanksgiving. Joe assembled the tree and checked to see that the lights were working, and I decorated it. Our two cats, Rascal and Simba, especially like to help with this annual project—jumping in and out of the tree storage box, exploring the ornaments before they're placed on the tree, and climbing into the tree, stretching out in the branches.

Every year during this time, Joe puts on his favorite Christmas music, Kenny G and Barbra Streisand. The recent Christmas was no exception. The snow on the ground and in the trees surrounding the house was visible through the three walls of windows in the sunroom. Joe would hum to the music and sing a little off-key with Barbra. He would dance a little and wiggle his hips as he picked up the tree sections and connected them together. Always a sight to behold. I was the clean-up crew of one and always tried to get Joe to be part of it, but it never worked.

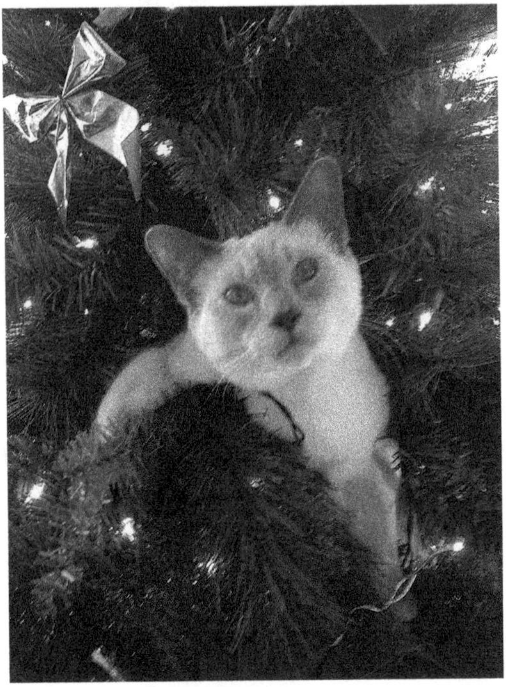

Between Thanksgiving and Christmas, I would shop for Joe and Greg. I would wrap presents as I purchased them, and gradually the Christmas tree skirt would be covered with gifts. It had become our custom to fly to Florida on Christmas Day or the day after and celebrate Christmas on Christmas Eve in Connecticut. In the aerospace industry, many companies are generally closed between Christmas Day and New Year's Day, so we had a week off. This year was no exception. Since Christmas was on Friday, we flew to Florida the following Sunday.

Greg had a few days off from work and drove home from Boston. We had our special Christmas dinner on Saturday: roast beef with horseradish sauce, twice-baked potatoes, salad, and green beans. I made Joe's favorite Christmas dessert—pecan pie and vanilla ice cream. After dinner, we sat in the sunroom and opened our gifts. Joe loves to try to have us open the presents in an "orderly" fashion. He also likes to pretend he's Scrooge and can do without Christmas. Not much chance of keeping things orderly, but he always had a pencil and paper and wrote down who gave him a gift so he could thank each person. When he would see my sisters or parents, he would be sure to thank them for whatever they sent him. And he always got it right, remembering who gave him each gift.

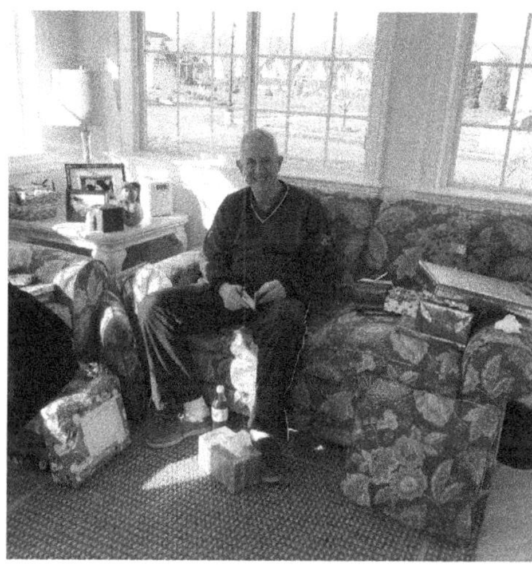

The nurse asks me if I'm okay, because I'm staring at Joe and trying so hard not to cry—I don't want Greg to see me break down. I ask when Joe will come out of the anesthesia, and she says it'll be morning before we can talk to him. I want to see him in a few hours and she says we can come back later, but not after 10 p.m. I don't want to be far away even though he's "sleeping."

It's around 3 p.m., and I haven't eaten yet today. Greg checks his smart phone to see what we can find in the hospital vicinity. Some restaurants aren't suitable for his vegan diet, but he finds a place he thinks will be okay. As we leave the hospital and walk out into the wind, I can't believe how cold it is. With the 13-degree temperature and the wind chill, it feels below zero. We're already numb from the inside out, so the temperature doesn't deter us. We aren't talking much —partly because of the cold and partly because we're both so worried. What is there to say?

The restaurant is on Cambridge Street, with a first-floor entryway leading underground. We place our order at the main counter and then find seats on one of the multiple levels. With our food balanced carefully as we sit, we both keep our eyes down, looking at our food.

Finally I say, trying to be cheerful, "It's such good news that the doctor said the surgery was a success! Your dad looked good, and he's getting really good care and attention in the recovery area. We'll see him again in a couple of hours." Then I ask him, "How are you feeling?"

Greg looks up at me and shrugs. "Dad looked pretty good. We'll have to wait and see how it goes."

I reach across the table, hold his wrist, and tell him, "He'll be fine. It'll take some time for him to recover, but he'll recover quickly."

Greg stares across the table and replies, "Mom, I hope so. Let's hear what the doctors tell us when we see them."

I change the subject and ask him about his work, his roommate, anything else....

We walk back to the hospital in the bitter cold. It hasn't warmed up in the least. I'm logistically disoriented, and I rely on Greg to find our way back to the hospital main entrance using the map app on his smartphone. We hang out in the waiting area, move my things to the car in the garage parking lot, and wait. We see Joe at about 5 p.m. and then have dinner in the hospital cafeteria in the Cox Building.

By the time we see him again at 9 p.m., his breathing tube has been removed and he very vaguely recognizes us. His voice is hoarse as he weakly acknowledges us. We approach his bed, I hold his hand, and Greg places his hand on his father's right shoulder. I tell Joe that everything went really well and that he's getting a lot of attention from the nurses. He smiles a little at this before he fades back into sleep.

The nurse tells us we can come back in the morning and that he'll likely be moved to a room sometime very early in the morning. I tell her I want to be with Joe when any doctors visit him, so she says I should go to his room by 7 a.m. She tells us a doctor stopped by while we were out and said everything looks normal. I'm disappointed that I missed the doctor. She gives me a phone number to the recovery area and tells me I can call anytime during the night to see how he's doing. She's very kind to us and tells us his recovery is going well and his vital signs are as they should be. I'm so exhausted, emotional, and tense. I don't want to leave Joe, but I can't stay in the recovery area all night, so I stay at Greg's apartment for the night.

Once we're at Greg's apartment, I call Joe's brother, Joe's sister, my parents, and my sister Peggy. I fill them in and tell them the surgery appears to be a success. They have a lot of questions that I can't answer, especially about how long Joe will be in the hospital. I have no idea at this point. I'm sleeping on the couch tonight, and after the phone calls, I fall into a restless, churning sleep. I call the recovery area at 2 a.m. and find out that Joe is doing well.

◆

The next morning, I wake up early and leave Greg's apartment at 6 a.m. It's very cold, around 20 degrees, but it's clear with little wind. Greg lives in Brookline, which is about four miles to the hospital. It can take 45 minutes or more to get to MGH, depending on traffic. I take Storrow Drive and exit on Government Center to Fruit Street. The navigation system calls out *Fruuuut Street* as Joe and I joked about a few days ago. Not so funny this morning without Joe in the car….

After parking in the car garage, I go the main entrance desk to find out where Joe is. They direct me to the 6th floor of the Lunder Building, where I eventually exit the elevator into the Herscot Atrium. I turn right, pass the waiting area on the left, walk through double glass doors, and stop at the nurses' desk to be directed to Joe's room. It's before 7 a.m., and I'm anxious to see Joe and any doctors who'll be coming by.

Joe is sleeping when I enter the room. He looks much the same as he did last night, but he doesn't seem to be as pale in the early dawn light. I'm crying and the day hasn't even started. How can this be happening? I sit down quietly and wait for a nurse or doctors to stop by. With all the waiting, I have plenty of time to think about Joe.

Although Joe and I met shortly after we both started working for the same company division, we didn't run into each other often. The company site had more than 20,000 employees, and the facility was very large. We were in different departments, and with so many social activities available, our paths didn't cross often. We had a mutual friend or two but were rarely at the same events. We were both learning our way around, building our knowledge base to support our careers. Joe took a couple of nine-month rotation assignments to East Hartford, and I left the company for a year or so and returned. It was several years later that we "remet."

> It's St. Patrick's Day in 1985, and I'm living in an apartment off the I-95 45th Street exit after the company rehired me. I've been back for a couple of months, and I'm planning to meet friends at Bennigan's for happy hour. They'll be serving green

beer for as long as it lasts, and a big crowd is expected. Beer kegs and an outside bar are set up in a roped-off area of the parking lot, which is packed with people.

At first I'm hesitant to go in, because I don't see my girlfriends anywhere and don't want to be pushed around by the crowd as I look for them. I hear someone call my name, and I turn around to see Joe with a man I don't know. Joe beckons me over—as one of the few women at our company, I'm easily recognizable. I'm relieved to see a familiar face. Joe introduces me to his brother, Jim, who's visiting from where he works in Louisiana.

We joke about the green beer, and Joe pinches me on the arm because he thinks I'm not wearing anything green. I point to the green earring I'm wearing, and I pinch him on the arm as payback. We talk about what's going on at work. When the two brothers start talking about playing golf—mostly rounds they played growing up—I make a few comments to let on that I also play a little. Joe talks about working at Oak Ridge Country Club and being a caddy for his father. He tells us about his father's "rules" for caddies—where they could stand, when they could move and talk, and so on. Jim laughs, as he's had the same experiences. What a fun time. I still can't find my friends, and I leave after talking to Joe and Jim for a while.

I decide I'll try to get together with Joe, because we seem to enjoy talking to each other. So I call him a week or so later. I'm nervous, as it isn't something I usually do. I identify myself and can tell he's surprised that I'm calling him. I tell him I'm taking my sailboat out on Saturday, and I ask if he'd like to join me. He pauses a little before telling me he can't go because he'll be playing golf that day.

I'm so embarrassed that I asked him, and I feel he's making an excuse to not go. After all, who would play golf with his buddies instead of going sailing with me? Not that I'm anything so special, but really? So I write him off, knowing I'll be able to find someone else to go sailing with me.

My musings are interrupted by the attending nurse coming in. Her name tag identifies her as nurse 'C', so I introduce myself. C appears to be in her late 20s or early 30s, and she speaks with a heavy Boston accent. She checks his fluid bags and changes one out. I ask her how he's doing, and she tells me he's been awake already. I'm surprised, but she explains that they want patients to be awake as soon as they're able and to be up and walking as soon as they can. Wow—just 24 hours ago, the surgery was starting.

Several doctors come into the room. I recognize the anesthesiologist, but I don't know the others. They quickly introduce themselves—all neurologists who want to see how Joe is doing. Joe wakes up, and I see him conscious for the first time since yesterday. The doctors ask him what day it is, and he knows it's Wednesday. They ask him what time it is, and he responds, "How should I know—where are my phone and watch?" They all smile at his response.

One doctor leans over Joe and shines a light into his eyes, then holds up his index finger and asks him to follow the finger with his eyes. Right, left, up, down…all good. Another doctor rolls a small object across Joe's left foot, then right foot, and asks Joe if he felt anything. His left leg was less responsive than his right. He asks Joe to close his eyes, then lift his left arm. He does, and it very gradually lowers. He's asked to do the same with his right arm; he lifts it and it stays in place.

Also, the left side of his smile is a little lower than the right. There are no hiccups. The doctors converse a little, and Joe interjects a question or two. He asks about the catheter, and they tell him it will possibly be removed later in the day. He asks if the compression boots can come off. "It feels like there are kittens kneading, getting ready to try to nurse on my leg," he says. They laugh, then tell him the boots can be taken off.

I ask about nausea, and they tell me he's on anti-nausea and anti-seizure medicines. He's also still taking steroids. All the medicines are being administered through his fluids. Today he'll try to drink liquids, then try eating food. In a day or so, they'll have him try get up.

I ask what to expect over the next days. They tell me Joe should regain his strength, followed by sitting up and walking. They think his thigh weakness should be better now that the tumor has been removed. When I ask about the weakness on his left side, they tell me that Joe's response is not unusual at this stage of recovery and that they'll be keeping an eye on it over the next few days. In a day or so, a physical therapist* and an occupational therapist* will come to assess how he's doing. I know Joe needs some time to recover, so I don't panic over any of the findings so far.

I'm allowed to stay in the hospital room during the day and overnight for the duration of Joe's stay. Nurses come see him regularly and help him with food, medicine, and getting up to go to the bathroom. There's never a period longer than two hours that there isn't a nurse or doctor coming to see him, and it's usually more frequent. It's difficult to sleep in the hospital with so many visits, but I know how necessary they are.

Doctors see him every morning and later in the afternoon. There's a doctor on call 24 hours a day, and the hospital doctor is available immediately if needed. Joe sleeps a lot, and when he wakes up, he's cheerful and chats with the nurses. He has his phone on his nightstand and checks it for texts from his friends, family, and work. He loves hearing from people.

A physical therapist and an occupational therapist work with Joe over the next few days. I can't believe how quickly they have him up and using a walker to get around. A few steps first, around the room next, followed by walking around the hallway and around the corridor—all within a couple of days. The weakness in his left leg is greatly diminished but not completely gone. The drooping on the left side of his mouth is much less noticeable. They keep a careful eye on his balance.

◆

On Friday, January 22, Dr N comes to visit Joe. We haven't seen him since the surgery. He inspects Joe's incision, which has been uncovered, and decides it looks as it should. He checks Joe's reflexes and eyes, has him stand and walk with the walker, and talks to him. He asks Joe what day and time it is, as does everyone else every time they enter his room. He checks Joe's left and right arm strength and continues to notice a slight difference between the two.

Dr. N tells us he's going to release Joe today, which takes me completely by surprise. Why so soon? The doctor explains how important it is that Joe not develop an infection after the surgery and that the best place for him to be to prevent such an infection is somewhere other than the hospital. He asks if we want to have Joe go to an assisted-care facility for the next couple of weeks. Since neither of us wants that, the doctor explains how careful we need to be at home to prevent infection, and he gives us instructions about when and how Joe can shower and wash his hair.

I ask about our two cats being around Joe. Dr. N is quite adamant that the cats should be nowhere near him until the incision has healed, which he expects will be in about four weeks. The staples will be removed in about ten days, and the additional pathology results should be available by then also. He tells us that around the time the staples are removed, we should talk with Joe's radiation oncologist* and neuro-oncologist* about follow-up treatment. Dr. N would like us to see him on February 18.

Dr. N explains that Joe will start tapering off the steroids and continue taking anti-seizure medicine, as well as resuming meds for other pre-tumor conditions. Greg comes to the hospital to help me with getting Joe home. He stays with Joe while I fill the new prescriptions at the hospital. Greg loads my car, and it's 4 p.m. by the time Joe is released. It's a Friday afternoon, so we decide we should drive home to Connecticut in the morning to avoid traffic leaving Boston.

Joe is so amazing. He laughs with his nurse C as he waits for the orderly to bring a wheelchair to take him to the hospital exit. She's a New England Patriots and Boston Red Sox fan, so over the last few days, he's been kidding her about the New York Mets winning the World Series. They commiserate about the Patriots not being in the Super Bowl this year. Joe tells her one of his favorite stories about the Boston Red Sox mascot, Wally the Green Monster.

"Hey, C, you aren't going to believe this. The Wally mobile was in our neighborhood over the Christmas holiday," he says.

She knows by now to be ready for the punchline from Joe, so she replies, "No way—you're just teasing me."

He says, "Really! And you can be sure my neighbors weren't happy about it. They're Yankee fans.

“And you know what else?” he continues. “It stopped and parked in my driveway!”

C looks at him blankly.

“And my son and his roommate got out of the car! Greg’s roommate Chris is Wally the Green Monster!” Joe explains that Chris is one of several people who are trained to perform at games and other functions. He got started after he was trained as a mascot for Boston University.

“And they really make some money doing this,” Joe adds, just as Greg comes into the room to catch the end of the conversation and corroborate his story. She doesn’t seem to be impressed, but I think she enjoyed the tale. Joe wasn’t trying to impress, he was just trying to share some info that she might get a kick out of. This is how he is with people—always trying to connect in a way they’d enjoy.

The orderly arrives with the wheelchair, and I thank C for all she’s done for us. She was truly a great nurse. I get the car from the parking garage while Greg stays with Joe so he can help him into the car. I’m surprised that Joe’s thigh strength appears better than it was before the surgery. He still needs some help getting into the car, though, especially to be sure he doesn’t bump his head.

Greg gets his car, and I follow him in my car to his apartment in Brookline. It takes close to an hour to get there, as we’re leaving at 4 p.m. to drive through Boston on a Friday afternoon. Once we get to Greg’s apartment building, he and I help Joe with his walker as we navigate up a slight incline to the entrance and then take the elevator to the second floor. Fortunately, Greg’s roommate is away, so Joe and I can stay in his room. I change the sheets, and we eat in. It’s an early night for us. I stay with Joe consistently to be sure he’s okay and to help with his medicines. He's taking so many that it's hard to keep them straight. Tomorrow is going to be a big day: we'll be going home.

Chapter 3: Getting Ready

"Hope" is the thing with feathers -
That perches in the soul -
And sings the tune without the words -
And never stops - at all -

Emily Dickinson

Today is Saturday, January 23, and I'm driving Joe home to Connecticut. After spending the night in Greg's apartment in Boston, I help Joe get ready for the trip home.

He needs help getting dressed, and I make him breakfast and give him his pills. I move things from the apartment to the car and make sure the sidewalk to the car has been salted and sanded to prevent ice. The last thing we need is for Joe to slip and fall. Just thinking about it gives me goosebumps of fear.

Joe is his usual affable self this morning, but I can tell he's nowhere near peak strength. His arms are tired when I help him with his shirt and pullover. I'm pleased to see he can stand up reasonably well, needing only a little assistance. He's using the walker around Greg's apartment and as we're leaving.

Greg is also coming to Connecticut to help his dad get settled at home. We're taking separate cars so Greg can return on Sunday to go to work on Monday. I'm so relieved that he'll be on the road with us, as I'm worried about Joe on the drive home. I put a clean pillowcase on the pillow Joe will use during the car ride home, vigilant to try to prevent wound infection.

Helping Joe down the walkway into the car is an experience as the walker bumps along the worn Chattahoochee pavers. Every bump makes me worry that it'll cause a balance issue for Joe. But it doesn't—he does just fine with me placing a guiding hand on the walker as he slowly makes his way to the car. He's being very cautious as we make our way downhill all the way to the car. We're very careful to make sure Joe doesn't bump his head when he gets into the car. The car is an Audi A6, which is a little low to the ground. But it's not too bad. Once Joe is situated with a pillow behind his head, seat partially reclined, and seatbelt on, we're ready to leave.

Greg takes the lead and we have our phones ready in case we need to talk on the way home. Joe closes his eyes to rest on the drive. This morning's preparation is a lot of effort for him. Not a word of complaint from him about anything, though. We start driving at around 9:30 a.m. I'm so glad we didn't try to leave late yesterday. The traffic isn't very heavy this morning, and there are very few trucks on I-90W as we drive along. It's about 30 degrees and a little overcast outside. We reach I-84W in about 80 minutes, then finish the trip home in another 25 minutes or so. Joe sleeps most of the way.

There are so many things I haven't thought of. For example, once I pull into our two-car garage, I realize there isn't enough room to use the walker to get to the side entryway door when there are two cars parked in it. So, I back Joe's car up to make room. There are two steps to get into the house, with no handrail for support, so we have to navigate the walker up a couple of stairs once we're inside the house. I'm so glad Greg is with us to help. Fortunately, we won't have to do this again until Joe is stronger. Joe shouldn't be in the main areas of the house until I've cleaned everything very well. Our two cats are free to roam anywhere in the house except the bedrooms, so Greg and I help Joe into the master bedroom on the first floor.

Greg stays with Joe while I relocate the cats, their litter box, and their food to the finished basement. The basement is an 800-square-foot area, so the cats should be fine there other than being lonely because they're separated from us. Rascal and Simba are excited to see me, purring and mewing as I pick them up to take them downstairs. I stay with them a while to make them (and me) happy. Rascal races me up the basement stairs as I leave, but I get to the door first. I feel awful closing the door and leaving them, but we're taking no risks of infection with Joe. I'll visit the kitties regularly during the day.

I clean the downstairs thoroughly and put a clean sheet on Joe's favorite recliner chair. We call it the *grog chair* because it's so comfortable that anyone who sits in it falls asleep. I set up a TV tray next to the chair so that anything Joe needs is close by. He was given an incentive spirometer* in the hospital to help keep his lungs healthy after surgery and was instructed to continue using it once every hour at home. He hates using it and says it's a form of torture, but I put it on the TV tray anyway—I'm going to insist he follow his doctors' instructions.

I then go to the grocery store and stock up on food. Joe has few dietary restrictions right now, so I look for all his favorites. Häagen-Dazs dulce de leche ice cream is on the top of the list. I'm grateful that Greg is here so I can leave Joe with him, but I'm afraid to leave Joe alone even though the grocery store is close by. I know I can go and get what I need and be back in under 30 minutes.

Once I'm home, I check on Greg and Joe. Joe is asleep, and Greg is watching a movie on his laptop. I think he's watching "The Hangover

Part II"—he likes to watch comedy movies. After Joe wakes up, Greg and I help move him into the living room and sit in the grog chair. He groans when he sees the spirometer.

Joe is alert, but naturally, he's tired. He's very cautious as he uses his walker to get to the chair. The large throw rug is a bit of an obstacle, so Greg and I roll it up and put it in the basement. We need to be sure that we eliminate any hazards to Joe getting around the house with the walker. The floors on the first floor are wood, and the only other throw rug is in the sunroom, so Greg and I move that rug to the basement too. Fortunately, the wood floors aren't highly waxed, so they're not slippery. And anyway, Joe is wearing his bright-yellow nonslip socks from the hospital–no need for fashion statements, and these socks are a real eyesore.

Now that the house is mostly set up, I feel more comfortable. There's been so much change so quickly that I haven't had much time to really think clearly. Joe's illness is the top priority, followed by the new house closing, the sale of the house in Jupiter, work obligations, financial and estate planning to finish… I feel my body tightening just thinking about everything I have to do.

I sit on the couch next to the Joe's chair. He has a long incision on the right side of his partially shaved head starting near his forehead and extending to his right ear. There are 33 staples in the incision to hold his skin taut and closed together. I stare at the incision and look for redness or swelling. I see none, but I'm not a nurse, so I hope I know what to look for.

Joe dozes in the grog chair while the TV above the fireplace is on. I also start to fall into a light sleep, knowing I'll be right next to Joe if he needs me. I'm so glad to be back in our house, away from the hospital and in a place I'm comfortable with. I didn't realize how exhausted and stressed I was until I start to relax. I know I won't be able to feel relaxed for long, but I seize the moment. Now that the surgery is over and we're home, I'm so hopeful about Joe's recovery. I'm also thankful that he's home from the hospital and appears to be following the anticipated recovery path.

I'm not confident about my knowledge about the recovery phase. It reminds me of the year Greg was born and how I felt bringing home such a tiny, totally dependent infant from the hospital. There were no instructions on how to care for a small baby, no guidance on how to bathe or feed him. But the love and fierce sense of protection a mother instinctively has for her child provided the intuitive base for sorting out how to nurture him. Now I'm feeling that same type of love and fierce protection for Joe, and I pray it'll help me do what's best for him as he recovers.

The hospital paperwork lists Joe's medications, and I have guidelines for which types of situations warrant calling the doctor's office. But the day-to-day maneuvering around the house, and the daily activities like showering, dressing, and using the walker, are all new skills that we need to develop and master. Joe appears to have full use of his legs, since the weakness on his left side is much less pronounced now. That's helpful when he uses his walker.

We both rest for several hours. I hear Joe stirring, and he says he needs to go the bathroom. I help him use his walker to get to the bathroom. Once we get there, we don't have any handrails for support, so we figure out how to use the walker for stability. That's one more thing we need to change in the house. At this point, I'm not sure if Joe will be using the walker temporarily or will need to use it long term. Right now, his balance doesn't seem to be a problem, and the weakness in his thighs continues to lessen.

I help Joe settle back into the grog chair before I make dinner. I was diligent in buying very healthy food, and I make a balanced meal of greens, meat, and starch—plus, of course, ice cream for dessert. I also bought a powder drink advertised to help with wound recovery. Because it's considered a supplement rather than a drug, it doesn't require review by the FDA.* So to be extra cautious, I had mentioned it to the doctor before we left the hospital and he said it was okay for Joe to have, though he didn't endorse the product. As we're finishing dessert, the front doorbell rings.

Greg's friend Colin arrives to visit him and Joe. Colin is Greg's longtime friend and a young man we're all very fond of. They met when they were both ten years old and starting middle school together. They shared many experiences in middle school and high school, and they maintained their friendship when they went to different colleges. They act more like brothers than friends and are constantly ribbing and teasing each other, but also helping each other with many situations. They both like to work out at the gym and have long used their workouts as a strategy to meet young ladies. They give each other advice on dating and other life situations, and it's very interesting and humorous to Joe and me.

Colin enters with a positive energy and enthusiasm that engulfs us all. "Hey, Mr. G! *So* glad to see you home from the hospital," he says as they do a fist bump. "Let me take a look at you. *Wow*, that's a long incision. It's really something. How are you feeling?"

"Couldn't be better," Joe replies. "You know there are 33 staples in my head?"

Joe smiles and looks at Colin. They talk about the surgery, the meds Joe is taking, and how he's feeling. Colin is in his second year of pharmacy school and has learned quite a bit about medicines. Then they start talking about how things are going with Colin's girlfriend. Colin explains that they're going through a little rough patch as she wants more of his time than he can give her because of his school requirements.

"Ah, just let her know who's boss and it'll be fine—don't let her push you around," Joe says with a wink.

Sage advice? Not exactly, but Colin laughs and goes upstairs to hurry Greg along so they can go to the gym. Before he leaves, I thank him for taking care of our kitty cats while we were in Boston and he tells me that he enjoyed spending time with them each day. I know how lucky we are that he helped us out and that he's our friend.

Joe retires for the evening at around 9 p.m. I help him with his walker a little, although he can manage it pretty well on his own. He needs help changing his shirt, as we want to be careful not to touch the incision when we're taking his shirt off or putting it on. I find a soft T-shirt that has buttons partially down the front for him to sleep in, and it's easier to put on than a typical men's polo shirt. I tell myself that going forward, I'll find casual shirts that button all the way down the front for him to wear during the day. We're very careful about washing his face and brushing his teeth. After he's propped up on pillows in bed, I lie down beside him until I can hear his steady and deepening breathing and I know he's asleep. Then I move into the family room, leaving the bedroom door open so I can go into the bedroom quickly if I hear any movement.

I call Joe's sister Jane, who wants to visit him. Jane lives in Colorado, two hours behind our time zone. Jane is a couple of years younger than Joe, and they have a typical sibling relationship. They do care for each other and share many common experiences.

"Hi, Jane; it's Lynn," I say when she answers the phone. "How are you doing?"

"Oh, I guess I'm doing okay," she replies. "Wondering how things are going with Joe. Can I talk to him?"

I explain that Joe is asleep and that I'm calling to make arrangements for her visit to Connecticut. I also tell her we're now home and that he's recovering as expected at this point.

"Jane, Joe will be recovering for the next four weeks or so," I tell her. "Everything here is focused on what he needs and how to help him regain his strength as soon as possible."

I explain that there are a lot of things to do to help Joe, including making his meals, helping him get dressed, keeping everything especially sanitary, and making sure he has plenty of rest.

"He's not really up to having guests, and he needs a quiet place where he can rest and relax, so I'm setting that up for him," I tell her.

"Well, I really want to see him as soon as I can. Is that okay?"

"Yes, it is," I reply. "But it'll be different from when you've visited before. Joe won't be feeling very well, and I'll be focused on how to help him. I'll be cooking things that he likes and they may not necessarily be what you can eat with your food allergies. You're welcome to be here, of course, but you'll need to handle your diet when you are here.

"Also, I won't be much of a hostess, and I'll ask that you help out by taking care of the room you stay in and clean up before you leave," I continue. "I'm sorry to ask this, but I can't do those things when I'm focused on Joe."

I explain that we'll be returning to Boston for appointments on February 3 and 4 and will be staying with Greg for at least one night. I warn her that Greg's apartment is small and she might have to sleep on the couch if she decides to come to Boston with us.

"I'm sorry, but that's what we have to do to help Joe," I conclude.

There's a long pause before Jane responds. "I've been looking for flights to Connecticut," she says. "I think I can be there sometime next week and stay for a couple of weeks. I understand what you're saying, and I'll bring some recipes with me so I can prepare some meals, and maybe you and Joe will want to have some of what I make. Would that be helpful?"

She also says she'd like to go to Boston so she can meet Joe's doctors. We agree that she'll finalize her flight arrangements and send me her itinerary.

I'm exhausted, and I go into the bedroom and sleep lightly next to Joe after I throw the sheets from the grog chair into the washing machine. I'm planning to wash and change the sheets every day to help reduce the possibility of infection.

◆

Joe is sound asleep when I wake up at around 6 a.m. on Sunday. I want to go to Mass this morning and then try to go to the gym to swim. Swimming has long been my exercise of choice to help manage stress from my job, and now I really need to go for a swim to help with the stress I feel about Joe's illness. I walk upstairs to Greg's room and wake him up. I ask him to sleep in our bed while I'm gone in case Joe wakes up and needs anything. I don't know how long Joe will sleep, but Greg very willingly agrees. It may not be necessary, but I really want to be sure that we watch Joe for any symptoms that may be of concern, such as breathing problems, and so Joe doesn't fall by trying to get out of bed by himself. I tell Greg I'll be gone until around 9 a.m.

It's in the 20s with a gusty wind this morning, but at least it's not snowing. The drive to the church is quite beautiful, with remnants of white snow in the evergreen trees and spread thinly on the ground, clean next to the brown tree bark. There are hardly any sounds, and there are very few cars on the road. I'm not completely over the extreme change we're dealing with, but I'm very focused on how to help Joe recover. There's no time to feel sorry for ourselves. I'm filled with hope that Joe will be that one-in-a-thousand case that will live a happy life for the next five years after surgery. The parking lot is slick with ice, and I take care walking to the front entrance of the church: small steps and short strides, since I see no salt or sand to help with traction. I sit in my usual pew and say a prayer to St. Jude, the patron saint of lost causes. Please, oh please, I beg, help Joe recover to his full potential….

I leave after Communion. Yes, I feel a little guilty about it, but I want to exercise and then get home as soon as I can. I'm lucky that there's a YMCA a few minutes from our house with a beautiful indoor Olympic-size pool. There are usually only a few people swimming and almost never any children in the pool on Sunday mornings. I find a lane and begin my laps. I've been swimming since my late 20s, and I have a routine that I follow. More often than not, I use this time to think about things and go into auto-swim mode. This morning, I think about what I've read about glioblastoma.

I know that once the growth is removed, what's most important is that it not start to regrow. So, a combination of radiation and chemotherapy is a common treatment option. The post-surgery treatment depends on the type of glioblastoma. When we go to Boston early next month, we'll find out what type Joe has. While I'm swimming, I pray that his glioma is treatable. But I know it's out of our control, so I decide to focus instead on what I can do to help him. I've been married to him for more than half my life, and I can't think about what life would be like without him. I'm determined that he *will* survive, and I have to find a way for him to live with dignity and happiness. I swim faster as I get more and more determined. We're not quitters—we're fighters, and Joe *will* be all right.

When I get home, I find Joe and Greg still asleep. Fine with me, as it can only be a good thing for Joe—lots of rest and quiet. I go to check on the kitties and spend some time with them. I think they know something is up because they're banished to the basement. They don't understand why they're here, and they're purring and so cuddly. It's very comforting to me, so I scoop them up and sit on the basement couch with them next to me. They meow over and over as I talk to them even though I know they don't understand a word I'm saying. I put on some soft music for them as I leave, and I hope it helps them a little. I'll be back in a few hours, and I know Greg will visit them today as well.

I prepare breakfast for Joe and have it ready to reheat when he wakes up. I hear sounds from the bedroom as I finish, so I know some activity is beginning. This morning will be Joe's first shower at home. I'm not sure exactly how we'll get it done—it depends on how he feels. I want him to eat first, but he wants to shower first. I take a deep breath and agree. It's a good sign to me that he wants to shower, but I'm not sure about his balance and strength.

We have a walk-in shower in the master bathroom—no bathtub. It's a small bathroom with the sink counter near the shower. The shower has clear glass doors that are firmly attached to the wall, with towel racks attached to them. I don't think these doors should be used for support, though. Okay, so how do we do this? Joe's incision shouldn't get wet for another few days, per the hospital instructions. I decide Joe can get into the shower with his back facing the showerhead, and then he can use a washcloth to wash himself as long as he doesn't lean over.

I pick out some clean clothes for Joe and put them on the bed before we try the shower. I put a clean nonslip shower rug on the floor against the shower and clean towels on the sink. The shower already has a nonslip surface, so we don't need an extra mat. Here we go. Clothes off in the bedroom first. Careful when removing the shirt to be sure not to touch the incision. Stand up and use the walker into the bathroom.

First problem: how Joe can get into the shower when the walker is in front of him. I move the walker to the right, and Joe holds it with his right hand—his stronger side. Thank goodness Greg is with us. He stands behind Joe, ready to hold him around the waist if necessary. I open the shower door and Joe steps in, with Greg very close to him.

Second problem: as I turn on the water, it's *so* cold at first. Joe yelps as it sprays on his back, and I quickly divert the spray to the shower wall until it warms up. Ordinarily, it might've been funny—but it's not so funny when we need to be sure Joe doesn't slip. Now the water is warm. Joe needs help using the washcloth, so I reach into the shower to help. Now it's my turn to yell as I get completely soaked reaching in. Too bad, but I can change later.

No water gets on Joe's head, and he's been cleaned all over. We turn the shower off and give Joe a towel. It's hard for him to dry himself off completely, so I help him. We position the walker so Joe can reach for it as he steps out of the shower. A short walk to the bedroom and Joe sits on the bed. I help him dress, and he's now ready to go to the family room for breakfast. The shower process took about 30 minutes, and I couldn't have done it without Greg for the first time. But I learned what I need to do differently, so next time will be easier.

Joe is hungry, and I'm absolutely thrilled that he wants to eat so much. Eggs, bacon, toast, orange juice, and sliced fruit for breakfast. He can't have caffeine, which means no diet soda. Breakfast of champions, plus lots of pills to take. Time for his favorite torture device, the spirometer. Joe wants to sit in the sunroom, so I put a clean sheet over the couch and give him pillows to rest his head on. With a full meal after so much effort from the shower, he closes his eyes and dozes off in the warm room. Greg joins Joe in the sunroom and keeps a watchful eye while I clean up from breakfast, change the sheets on the master bedroom bed, and wash clothes. I'm a fanatic about keeping everything clean to prevent the incision from becoming infected.

I'm taking full advantage of Greg being with us today. He'll go to Boston tonight, so while I have the chance, I get as much done as I can. I call my sister Peggy to talk about how things are going.

I'm the middle daughter of three, and Peggy is my younger sister by four years. She's not only my sister but someone I'd have as a friend even if we weren't related. Her husband Mike and Joe became friends over the years through sharing many family events. They're both very concerned about Joe.

I start the conversation with my usual perfunctory opening: "Hi, Peggy; it's Lynn. How are you doing?"

"We're fine here," she replies. "How are you and Joe?"

"Well, we came home from the hospital yesterday. Joe was released Friday," I say. "I can't believe the doctors sent him home so soon. They told us he was better off recovering somewhere other than the hospital."

Peggy tells me that Mike's doctors did the same after his surgery because they were concerned that he might contract something that'd make his weakened state even worse if he stayed in the hospital.

"Anyway, it's quieter here, and I think I can make sure Joe has better food to eat and gets a lot of rest," I say. "It helps to be in a familiar place without all the constant visits from doctors and nurses, even though it made me feel secure knowing they were constantly checking on him."

I tell my sister how worried I'm that, because I don't have any training, I might miss signs of a problem and won't call Joe's doctor when I ought to.

"I feel so uneducated, and like I'm floundering," I continue. "I'm doing what I think I should do, but I don't know if what I do is right."

Peggy tells me that if I was given instructions with the discharge papers, they ought to tell me what to look for.

"I did receive instructions, but I'm still concerned," I tell her.

We talk a little about it and about all the things I need to do in addition to taking care of Joe. I'm completely overwhelmed by how Peggy responds.

"Lynn, I want to help you with your homes in Florida if I can," she says. "If you'll let me, I can represent you at the closing of your new house in February. And I can move things from the house in Jupiter to the new house once the older house is sold."

I haven't figured out how to deal with the house closing, particularly the walk-through of the house before the closing. Paperwork, legal services, and finances can be handled long distance, but making sure the house is acceptable to buy requires that someone be there in person. I'd been considering asking Greg to stay with Joe while I flew to Florida for a day or so to take care of things.

So when Peggy makes her offer, the relief I feel consumes me. But I also feel weak that I'm thinking of letting her do all that for me. Peggy still has a lot on her plate, as Mike's surgery for throat cancer was about sixteen months ago. Mike and Peggy still go to Baltimore four times a year for checkups to test Mike's progress. So far, so good, but it's far from a clean bill of health. I haven't relied on anyone other than Joe for many years, and I don't know how to accept help from others. But I realize that this is an extraordinary time and that I need to seriously consider Peggy's offer. We talk about how it could work without affecting the things she needs to take care of.

"Lynn, I really want to do this for you," she insists. "I can't come to Connecticut and help you there, but I can manage this. That way, you can be with Joe."

Peggy tells me she can drive to the east coast in a few hours, complete the home inspection, and sign the necessary documents if I give her power of attorney. She has bought and sold a few homes and understands what to check, but she says I can give her a list of anything else I'd like her to look for.

I feel so guilty and indebted accepting her offer. But I'm confident she'll do it well, and I know how much it'll help us. Joe and I don't want his remaining time to be spent in Connecticut when we could have a few good years enjoying each other in a better climate and in a place we both love, so we plan to move to Florida as soon as he's healthy again. Joe so wants to return to work, and we hope he'll be allowed to work from Florida. Peggy's proposition is the first step of that course. I feel so fortunate that she's my sister and friend, and I'm so grateful for her offer of help. Joe and I are in a terrible situation, and

I cry quietly knowing how blessed I am to have help offered that I wouldn't have thought to ask for.

Joe relaxes for a while before we have lunch. A couple of hours later, my cell phone rings. I don't recognize the number, so I almost let it go to voicemail. But I'm so glad I decide to answer it, because the voice on the other end is offering us some help.

"Hello, may I please speak to Joseph Gambill?" the caller says.

"This is Lynn, his wife," I respond "Can I help you?"

The caller, whom I'll call "C," explains that she works for a local nursing agency referred by MGH. She tells me Joe must give her permission to talk to me, so I hand the phone to him and he gives his okay. C tells me that as follow-up to Joe's surgery, she'll come to our house to check his wound and vital signs and evaluate what other home care he should have. She says she'd like to come tomorrow, and I'm so happy that I can't agree fast enough. We make arrangements for her to come at 10 a.m. on Monday, and I give her directions to our home. It's such a relief to me. I thought I'd be taking care of Joe on my own until his next appointment in Boston. Having an RN see Joe in our home is too good to be true. I decide to check with our insurance company to be sure it's allowed, and ultimately, the service is covered and approved! I so welcome this much-needed help! This truly has been a day of good news for us as we try to navigate forward.

Greg leaves for Boston in the late afternoon. I'm always sorry to see him leave, but I'm especially apprehensive because I'll be taking care of Joe myself, alone, for the first time since his surgery. Joe is tired, but he can clearly communicate, is eating well, and can walk with his walker without losing his balance. He's also following instructions, like taking his pills and even using the spirometer he hates, and he's very careful getting around. He has no difficulty speaking and is showing no obvious mental changes since the surgery. It's so hard to tell at this point if there are any changes, which seems like a great sign for an untrained person. He doesn't slur his speech, he recognizes people he knows, and his left leg, arm, and face appear similar to his right. He's very tired, as I expected. After all, he just had a seriously major surgery. My goal is to help him become stronger every day so he can return to all the things he loves to do. I'm not comfortable leaving him alone, which is one of the many things I'll talk to the nurse about tomorrow.

The day continues to be a quiet one for us. We have an early dinner and watch a little TV before Joe retires for the evening at around 9 p.m. I help him brush his teeth, wash his face, change his clothes for bed, and get propped up on pillows. He needs to sleep on his back, not on his side. I get in bed and rest next to him until I hear his deep steady breathing and know he's asleep. Then I return to the TV room, leaving the door open behind me so I can hear any movement from the bedroom.

Using my tablet computer, I create a list of questions for the nurse. How does she think he's doing? Is the wound okay? Are his breathing, blood pressure, and heart rate okay? Does he have a fever? Is there any special food that will help him recover faster? Is the amount of sleeping normal? What about possible seizure? I've noticed he gets a little bit confused about the pills he needs to take. Before the surgery, Joe was responsible for taking his medicine himself. Now he gets a little confused with the schedule, even with the updated spreadsheet I prepared. Is that normal? (I think it is, considering he just had major brain surgery.) What would she expect his recovery time to be? How do I monitor his progress to understand if he's recovering as he should be? I'm sure there are more things I should ask, but I don't know what they are. You don't know what you don't know.

I'm anxious, and I feel foreboding in my heart. I don't know why. I suppose it's seeing Joe with the very long incision in his head. And seeing that he's so tired. I know it's to be expected, but it's such a recent change. Joe has had his share of health issues over the years, but they've always been manageable. This is very different. My emotions are up and down. Hope and then anxiety. And this overwhelming need for him to recover. I feel so helpless and powerless to change what's happening. So, I keep finding things to do, like cooking, cleaning, doing laundry, getting Joe's clothes ready—anything to feel useful. Most important, being patient and showing love for Joe. I think that there may be something a little different about Joe now, but I can't be sure if it's because he's just tired.

◆

Monday morning starts with our day-old routine. Before Joe wakes up, I replace the sheets on the grog chair and the sunroom couch. I then cook breakfast and have it ready to be warmed up when Joe is ready to eat. He's still asleep, and I have no intention of waking him. He'll wake himself up when he's ready. It's still early, around 8 a.m. I notice that my wedding ring isn't on my finger. Ah, yes—I put it away because I didn't want it to scratch Joe when I was helping him use the walker, shower, or change clothes. It's such a beautiful ring, and I hate to not wear it. It's not my original wedding ring. It reminds me of how Joe and I began dating, especially when I never thought we would actually go out. So I start reminiscing about our time in Florida.

> The phone rings in my apartment. It's a landline, and I race across the room to answer it. I suspect it's a call from work, as I'm on call this evening.

"Hello, this is Joe Gambill. May I speak to Lynn?" a soft-spoken southern voice asks.

I hesitate a moment, remembering our last conversation. I could pretend I'm a roommate and tell him Lynn isn't home. But that would be the cowardly way, so I quickly abandon the thought.

"This is Lynn," I reply. "What, not playing golf tonight? Moonlight golf or something else?"

Joe laughs in response.

"Well, if I could've found a foursome, I probably would be," he says. "But all the lights are out on the course tonight, so I thought I'd give you a call."

"Second choice, I see," I reply. "Well, maybe you should call me when I'm the first choice."

I suppose that's a bit direct, but let's be clear where we stand. Now it's Joe's turn to hesitate.

"All kidding aside, I was thinking I'd like to take you out to dinner this weekend," he says. "There's a new restaurant, Panama Hatties, that's supposed to have really great food. Would you like to have dinner Saturday night?"

"I've heard it's a good restaurant, and yes, I'd like to go. Thanks for asking," I respond.

Joe asks where I live and suggests he pick me up at 7:30 p.m. After I give him directions, we talk a little about how things are going at work. Then we're off the phone after a short conversation. I'm surprised that he called. And I'm surprised that I agreed to go.

> Our first date is so much fun. Joe is on time, opens the door for me (you'd be surprised how this is practically a lost art), and has made a reservation with a view of the inlet waterway. He's so pleasant to the restaurant staff, including the maître d', the servers, and our waitress. There's none of that "I'm better than you because I'm the patron of the restaurant" stuff, which is a big turnoff for me. Just the right amount of conversation with each person to be sure they knew he's a regular guy. We talk about sports, including football and golf. Joe graduated from the University of Tennessee and continues to be an avid fan. When he finds out I went to the University of Georgia, instant ribbing begins—but in a funny way, not derogatory. Joe learned to play golf a little later in age than I did, and we talk about recent golf tournaments. Jack Nicklaus, Curtis Strange, Ben Crenshaw, Lee Trevino, Greg Norman…*and* Jack Nicklaus lives in Palm Beach Gardens! Sooner than later, we talk about handicaps and playing golf together. We agree to play next weekend to see who'll have the best round using our handicaps. To make it interesting, we bet that the loser has to buy dinner at the winner's restaurant of choice. We move on to the topics of music, movies, work, common friends, and other things people talk about when they're getting to know each other better. Conversation is easy, and we're both having a good time. You can tell when things are clicking….

Now, as I look at my ring finger, I wonder how we've come so far. We've been married 28 years—almost half my life. We dated for about two years before we got married in 1988.

> One day in June 2013, Joe calls me at work. We often go out to eat after work, especially if we're both working late. We have a

few local favorites, and tonight we agree to meet at Bellini's in South Windsor. As we finish dinner, Joe takes my left hand in his. He looks me in the eye and says, "We have an anniversary coming up. It's bccn almost 25 years since we were married."

His fingers roll the wedding ring on my finger as he continues, "I'd like to go shopping with you this weekend so we can pick out a new ring for you. I love you so much, and I don't know how you've put up with me all this time." And he leans over and kisses me.

I don't know what surprised me more—that he remembered our anniversary, that he wanted to buy me a new ring, or that he'd go shopping with me. It was such a special evening for us. It meant everything to me that he wanted to do all of that. After all the time we were married, he was trying to do something that he thought meant something to me. But what meant more to me was his thoughtfulness—that he wanted to do that for me and that it was his idea. Now, the ring I put away is the one Joe and I picked out together for our 25th anniversary.

I go into our bedroom to check on Joe and see that he's starting to move around a little. I sit on the side of the bed and watch him. He's propped up on pillows, as he's sleeping on his back. He knows not to sleep on either side, and he seems to be reasonably comfortable. Just as I decide that he really isn't ready to wake up, his eyes open. He looks around and then stares at me. I ask him how he feels, and he gives me his standard answer—"fine." Oh, really, I think—seven days since brain surgery and you're fine? I think not. He says he had some really strange dreams about his parents, and he tells me how much he misses them. And his eyes tear up. I tell him how much his parents love him and that they're always with him, helping him. I hug him and hold his hand while he talks about his mom and dad.

After a few minutes, Joe tells me he wants to get up. I ask him if he wants to shower or eat first, and he says he'd rather eat. I think that's a good idea, as I want to be sure he's strong enough for his shower. He needs help getting dressed, particularly so he doesn't lean over to put clothes on. He uses his walker to go to the dining room table while I walk behind him to help if he shows any signs of instability. He's walking carefully and shows no balance issues.

Joe has a good appetite and eats a large breakfast. Today it's blueberry pancakes, bacon, fruit, and orange juice. No diet soda, as he still can't have caffeine. He rests a little after breakfast, and then we decide to try a shower. I'm nervous because it'll be the first time I'm helping him shower without Greg's help. Based on yesterday's trial run, I decide to get in the shower with Joe so I can help if he has any balance issues and help with washing. So I put on a bathing suit and shower cap—yes, looking my loveliest—and help him walk to the shower. It goes better than yesterday, as we know what to do with the walker. I turn the water on first to get it warm, and I put nonslip bathroom mats all the way around the shower doors. Joe steps into the shower first, with me right behind him. I help him turn so his back is facing the shower, like yesterday. It works out pretty well, and we manage to keep Joe's wound free of water. Next I help him step out of the shower, get dried off, and walk into the bedroom to sit on the bed. After he's dressed, I help him walk to the sunroom. Not quite a half-hour process, but it's still fatiguing to Joe. He rests on the couch in the sunroom with the warm sun streaming in. While he rests, I go change my clothes and clean up the towels and mats in the bathroom.

We have about an hour until the visiting nurse, C, arrives. I don't know what to expect, but I'm so happy that someone is coming to evaluate Joe. I clean up from breakfast and vacuum the TV area. No infection from this house.

When C arrives, she explains that her role is to evaluate Joe to determine the extent of home care he should have. She says she'll check his vital signs and his wound and that she wants Joe to answer her questions himself so she can determine his current level of capability.

C washes her hands in our kitchen sink and then puts on sterile gloves. I take her to the sunroom to meet Joe. Before she begins her evaluation, she has Joe sign several forms, including a permission form allowing her to talk to me about his health. Then she examines his incision and tells us that it looks clean, with no unusual redness or swelling that might indicate infection. She asks if he has washed his hair yet and tell her weren't supposed to yet, but she looks over the paperwork and says we should do so tomorrow. Uh-oh, I wonder to myself—how are we going to do this? She checks his temperature and blood pressure and then has him use the dreaded spirometer. All good, and I'm so relieved.

Next, C has Joe close his eyes while he's seated and has him extend both arms in front of him. She tells him to keep his arm tight while she pushes down on each arm. The right arm stays in place, but the left arm is weaker. She performs a similar activity with his thighs and gets the same result—his left isn't as strong as his right.

She then has Joe stand up and show her how he uses his walker. He's very careful using the walker—not unsteady, but not confident, either. She asks him to stand and close his eyes. Standing behind him in case he needs support, she evaluates whether he sways and, if so, how much. She then has him sit again while she asks him basic questions, like the date, the day of the week, his age, and when he was born. He doesn't know the date—but to be fair, neither do I.

C tells us that an RN will come to the house every other day and that she's going to send a physical therapist and an occupational therapist to work with Joe. How long they'll work with him depends on his progress, but it will initially be for ten visits each. Then there'll be another evaluation to assess his needs. Before she leaves, she tells us both therapists will contact me today to schedule appointments and one should be coming tomorrow. I feel so much better knowing she has checked on Joe.

I decide that I need to follow up with our insurance carrier to be sure that what C recommends is approved. I've called the insurance carrier a couple of times since Joe's diagnosis and surgery. Every time I call our insurance carrier, it's a hassle. I always have to start with an 800 number, and then an automated phone system would tell me to "listen carefully to the menu items, as they have recently changed." The phone system asks for a Social Security number, a case number, and the reason for my call. It doesn't offer an option that's relevant to my reason for calling. Back to the main menu. I continually repeat that I want to speak to a representative. Finally, I'm put on hold for a representative. I typically wait 15 to 45 minutes for an actual person to speak to. Once a representative answers, they won't speak to me without Joe's permission. So I bring the phone to him and he gives permission. I ask them to put the permission in his file so that I don't have to go through the same thing again every time I call. They say they will, but I'm skeptical. I finally get confirmation that the nurse and therapist visits are approved. I ask that the approval be mailed to me, because I plan to keep a copy of all approvals to avoid billing problems later.

Handling the business aspect of Joe's illness is stressful and frustrating, but I know it has to be done accurately. The last thing I want is for my stress to flow over to Joe, so I try to keep myself in check dealing with it. But I'm not always successful.

The rest of the day is similar to the previous day. Lunch, rest, quiet music, a little bit of walking with the walker, dinner, early bedtime. Jane called to tell us her travel plans: she'll be arriving Thursday and staying for 11 days.

◆

On Tuesday and Wednesday, we follow a similar routine, except that I help Joe wash his hair during his shower. The first day is very challenging. I use baby shampoo because I'm afraid soap suds will sting his eyes. He's not supposed to lean his head down when we rinse his hair because it could make him lose his balance.

So, after I follow Joe into the shower, I put a little shampoo in my hands and carefully put it on the top of his head, away from the incision. I massage the shampoo into his hair and let the water from the showerhead flow slowly over the incision and staples. Joe has his eyes closed, and I hold his arm to help stabilize him if necessary. Once the shampoo is rinsed out, I reach behind him and turn the shower off. I quickly grab a towel and gently dry his face off so he can open his eyes. Then I help him completely towel dry. We then finish our shower routine, including using the walker to step away from the shower and getting dressed.

The physical therapist comes to our house on Tuesday. After she conducts an evaluation, she provides a daily exercise program to help

Joe improve his strength, walking skills, and balance. The physical regimen includes exercises he should do when he's seated and then some walking without his walker. Joe should do the exercises twice a day and walk at least three times a day. He's very willing to do so, because he knows it will help him regain capability. He'll have physical therapy two or three times a week, and the plan will be modified as he improves.

The occupational therapist visits on Wednesday. She focuses on Joe's comprehension skills and on his ability to care for himself and complete daily activities—what she calls activities of daily living, or ADLs—like eating, preparing food, getting dressed, personal grooming, showering, reading, and managing his own medicine. She also recommends we purchase an adjustable shower chair, grip bars to mount on the shower wall, a different walker, and a raised toilet seat.

Both the physical and occupational therapists check Joe's vital signs before they start to work with him. They also conduct many of the same tests that the registered nurse did on her initial visit. Both scrupulously wash their hands immediately upon entering the house and before leaving and provide definitive plans and helpful recommendations for Joe.

As with the registered nurse visit, I feel immense relief with the therapists' visits. We have "homework" to do. Great—focus areas to help Joe get better! I'm happy to comply with all their recommendations. Each therapist will see Joe twice a week initially. One of my jobs is to help him complete the assignments.

I'm very excited that we have focused plans, and I believe they'll be very helpful. Joe and I both feel we're in good hands and are being provided guidance so Joe will improve quickly.

The therapists visit from 10 a.m. to 11 a.m. Joe is usually so exhausted afterward that he naps in the sunroom for a couple of hours until we continue with our newly defined routine.

The therapist visits aren't the only things going on during the day. Before the surgery, Joe was basically addicted to his phone messages, texts, and emails. That hasn't changed. Joe's phone is next to him wherever he is, except in the shower. It's like a lifeline to him. Coworkers, friends, and relatives text him, and he lets them know what's happening. His texts are coherent for the most part, but he occasionally gets the texts mixed up and sends responses to the wrong person. It doesn't happen often, but when it does, it's usually later in the day as he gets tired.

While we were away for Joe's surgery, various communications had arrived in the mail. There are many get-well cards for Joe, which he loves seeing. There are also various documents for insurance, bills, and financial information. It's obvious that addressing them isn't within Joe's current capability, so they fall to me to take care of. Joe has long taken care of our home bill payment structure, and I now find myself taking charge of it. It's very difficult, because much of the information is set up on the computer with passwords that only Joe knows. Or knew, I should say. That's when I start to worry that things are a little different. Joe has always had a fantastic memory, but now he doesn't remember passwords and doesn't know his way around our home computer. I begin resetting log-in credentials and doing whatever else is required. But I'm worried about Joe's short-term memory, and I hope he'll eventually regain it.

I know very little about the function of various parts of the brain. I know Joe's tumor was in the right frontal lobe. As I research the frontal lobes, I learn that lesions in that area can cause a wide variety of symptoms, including issues with motor function, problem solving, spontaneity, memory, language, initiation, judgment, impulse control, and social behavior.* There it is: *memory*. I'm reserving my concerns for a few more weeks to see if the change in his short-term memory is really a product of recovering from surgery or a longer-lasting effect.

◆

Thursday, January 28, is the first day Joe is supposed to follow his new exercise routine. And Joe's sister Jane is arriving this afternoon. We start our day as we usually do: breakfast, shower, rest—oh, wait…now we have to complete the exercises twice a day, and walk around the house without the walker, if possible. That means rest time is shortened to about 45 minutes. I then cajole Joe into doing his exercises.

Joe knows how important the exercises are, but it's another thing to actually do them. He's an avid golfer, but he has never loved to exercise. He usually makes a New Year's resolution to go to the gym and sticks with it for six to eight weeks. Here we go, starting an exercise program at home, and Joe needs some inspiration to start.

I set up a chair for the exercises he needs to be seated for. The side of the kitchen counter is the most stable location for the few exercises that require standing. I clear space off the counter so Joe can hold on as needed.

"Joe, are you ready to try these new exercises?" I ask him.

"Yes, I'm ready," he replies.

But there's no movement from the couch in the sunroom. I wait a few minutes and ask again. Same reply. Okay, this isn't going to work, I think to myself. So I go into the sunroom, hands on my hips.

"Come on, Joe, let's do this," I say.

He looks at me and says okay. But still no action. I put the walker in front of him.

"Okay, ready now?" I ask.

Still he says yes but doesn't move. I go and sit next to him.

"Joe, are you going to do this or not?" I ask him.

He turns his head to me, sighs, and says, "I want to. But I know how hard it's going to be. I know I need to, but it's going to be difficult."

I really feel for Joe now, as it's so unlike him to admit that something is difficult. It's totally out of character for him, so I know he isn't confident that it'll be worth the effort.

"Joe, this is going to help you so much," I tell him. "You'll get stronger every day if you do it. I know how much you want to go back to work. But you can't right now, because you wouldn't be able to get around. How could you get from the parking lot into the building, or take the stairs to your office, or walk from meeting to meeting like you used to do?

"I'll help you with the exercises, and I'll do them with you," I reassure him. "Together we'll get really good at it, and you'll see how much better you'll feel. Will you try it with me? The hardest days will be the first couple, and then you'll get stronger so quickly!"

Joe is studying my face and eyes while I talk with enthusiasm. I do believe this will help him! He puts his hands on the walker handles, pulls himself to a standing position, and pushes the walker to the chair I set up.

The exercises are fairly basic, but they're hard for Joe to do. I sit in a chair next to him and do them with him. I try to get him to count the repetitions out load as some motivation. I'm surprised that he has trouble counting to ten out loud and mixes up the numbers, so I start counting with him. I think it takes him a lot of concentration to do the exercises, let alone count them at the same time. We do the exercise slowly, and I encourage him along the way. I can see he's really trying. We finish most of the exercises and then decide that's enough for now, so I help Joe back to the couch. I feel it was a good first effort. The more we do it, the easier it will be for him.

While Joe rests, I sit on the sofa in the TV room. I can see him in the sunroom and can hear his breathing. I cry softly as I remember the golfing date we had a bet on many years ago. And I remember all the times we used to jog together, Joe always being the stronger runner, racing me as we would finish and of course finishing first.

> Our golfing date was the first of many times we played golf together before Greg was born. It was the summer of 1986, and we played at Deer Creek in Delray Beach using the Lung Card, a charity initiative by the American Lung Association that offers discounts at golf courses. We both played the men's tees, and it was clear that Joe was the stronger player. But around the green, we were somewhat equivalent, and I was the better putter. We weren't very poorly matched, but Joe had a better overall game than I did. So he won the round, even with our handicaps accounted for. Before we started the match, we had agreed that the loser would treat the winner to dinner and drinks at Café Du Parc in North Palm Beach, the most expensive restaurant in our area. You can be sure that there was lots of heckling from Joe after he won. We agreed that we'd go to the restaurant the next weekend.

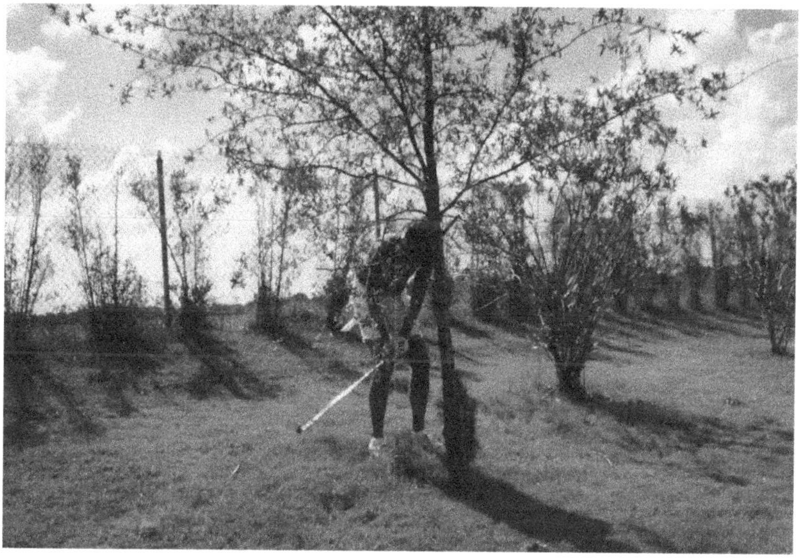

It's Saturday night—the night of our dinner date—and the earliest reservation I could get was 9 p.m. Joe is chivalrous enough to drive, so he picks me up at around 8 pm. He's planning to make the most of having dinner and drinks on my tab. The restaurant is very crowded while we wait at the bar. Once we move to our table, we both spare no expense on our orders. It's a five-course meal including dessert, and we eat for close to two hours. When the bill arrives, I signal the waiter to give it to me. Joe watches carefully for my reaction to the bill.

"Oh my Gosh, you really know how to spend the money, don't you?" I exclaim jokingly. "This is my whole paycheck! I won't be able to eat all next week. I better get a doggy bag!"

The bill is over $175, which is quite expensive, but I'm deliberately exaggerating the impact for effect. He tries to take the bill from my hand to see the damage, but I won't let him. I pay the bill, and he keeps asking me how much it was. I never did tell him the cost, even after 28 years of marriage. It was a running joke with us that would come up periodically while we were married, as he would ask me again about the bill. I did learn to never bet against Joe in golf again, though.

Now, looking at Joe on the sofa in the sunroom, I pray that he'll become strong again. His face is relaxed as he sleeps, but his complexion is a bit wan. He breathes deeply and has a pillow on his stomach, with one arm resting on the pillow. To look at him, you'd think he's older than he is. He's 58 years old, and his hair is almost white gray. He has a lanky build but has put on a few pounds gradually over the last several years. He weighs about 190 lbs. and has a soft, slightly protruding belly. At 6'3", he's tall enough to carry extra weight without it showing very much. He has the most beautiful smile I've ever seen—positively mischievous, but kind. And he flashes that smile often. Even though he's unwell, he usually smiles at the nurse and therapists as they work with him. He's not one to complain or grumble.

It's now close to 3:30 p.m., and I'm expecting Joe's sister to arrive at any time. Fortunately, she's renting a car at the airport and driving to our house once her flight lands. She's flying out of Denver, although she lives in Boulder. I'm looking forward to her being here, as I hope she can help Joe and me. Jane arrives close to 4 p.m., and Joe is now sitting up in the sunroom. I greet her at the door and help her with her luggage. Then I show her to Greg's bedroom, where she'll be staying. It's on the second floor and has a full bathroom and adjoining den area. Basically, the upstairs of the house is hers to use as she needs.

Jane then joins Joe in the sunroom. They don't look alike, and I don't think anyone would think they're related. Jane wears her thick curly hair shoulder length. As both of her brothers have experienced themselves, her hair has grayed over the years. She's diminutive in stature and dresses in garb similar to a college student, often in gray, blue, or black.

Joe looks at Jane as she enters the sunroom. “Hey, sister, what do you know?” he says.

“Well, not too much, now that you ask,” she replies. “Let me take a look at you, big brother. Whoa, that it is some impressive doctoring I see evidence of. How are you feeling?”

Pointing his finger at me, Joe says he’s feeling “middling to good” except for the torture I put him through with the exercises we did in the morning. Jane follows the finger pointing to me and gives me a questioning look. Uh-oh, I think—she doesn’t know he’s supposed to be doing the exercises and probably believes I’m hurting him. I decide I’ll fill her in later. Joe and Jane catch up a little, and he tells her about the surgery and how he feels. She fills him in a little on what she’s been doing. After an hour or so, she decides to go to the grocery store. I give her directions, as it’s close by and easy to find.

While she’s gone, Joe and I eat our dinner and continue with our routine. Throughout the day, Joe has been consistently answering e-mails from friends and colleagues. He regularly communicates with Jean and Mike. They’re work colleagues and friends who care very much about Joe. They tell him they want him to recover and come back to work as soon as possible. Joe also has his phone set up so it sends him the latest news on sports and current events. Over dinner, he mentions several items of interest to him that he read from his phone. Joe tells me he feels bad that he’s missing work now, because January and February are very busy months.

We set our business objectives and goals for the year and complete end-of-year goal evaluations. Joe is key to developing and communicating these goals to his team, and he feels responsible for completing the task. But he understands that being out of the office means that the duty should be delegated.

Jane returns from the grocery store as Joe and I finish our meal. It's good timing in that I can quickly clean up and leave her to the kitchen to prepare what she wants to eat. Joe retires to the grog chair, and Jane talks to him while she cooks. I coordinate with my sister Peggy on the home sale she's completing for us, making her copies of information and preparing it to be mailed.

The next day, after breakfast and Joe's shower, I prepare for his exercises. This time I set up two chairs side by side and lay the exercise sheets on the kitchen counter. I explain Joe's homework to Jane, and she says she wants to participate, so I add a third chair. Joe is showing a little more interest in doing the exercises today. Using his walker, he guides himself to the chair in the middle and sits down. I sit on his left, Jane on his right. I describe the first exercise sheet and we proceed. I think Joe will have a little fun "leading" us in the exercises, so I ask him to count out loud. He does okay for the first few but then gets confused with the count, so I help him.

Joe needs encouragement to finish all the required work, but I'm thrilled to see that he does it all. Joe is really happy with the praise he's getting from us both. Now, Joe is no child, but the exercises are hard for him after the surgery he has had. You catch more bees with honey… Also, since the surgery, things have been changing in his brain that affect his motor control. In addition to the concentration it takes to do the exercises, he's in a weakened state, so feeling that he's accomplished something meaningful is important.

Over the next couple of days, the RN and both therapists return. Each tells us Joe is progressing and doing well. There are no signs of wound infection, and he's holding his own on strength building. M, the physical therapist, makes a few modifications to the exercise routine and adds a few others, and this interests Joe a little. He feels stronger and is a little more confident in moving around the house. He's even initiated the exercise routine himself a couple of times instead of me coercing him into it. Jane is helping by cooking a couple of meals in the evening and keeping Joe company during the day. This frees me up to run errands and to exercise at the gym a little. Both therapists tell me I need to keep my strength up while I'm caring for Joe. After all, how can I take care of him if I'm not healthy myself?

Soon we're approaching Joe's two-week post-surgery appointments at MGH. He has an MRI and visits with several doctors scheduled for February 3 and 4. We're planning to stay with Greg the evening of the 3rd and then return to Connecticut on the 4th. Jane wants to go to Boston with us, so I again explain the sleeping situation in Greg's apartment. I tell her she'll most likely have to sleep on the couch since there's not an extra bedroom. Joe and I will stay in Greg's room and Greg will sleep on a pull-out couch in his roommate Chris's room since Chris won't be traveling. It'll be "cozy." Chris is so gracious to agree to these accommodations. Greg wants us to stay with him to optimize the time he can spend with us.

◆

As I get us ready to leave on Wednesday morning, Joe and I discuss our plans. I explain whom we'll see and when we'll see them, and Joe acknowledges that we'll find out more from the pathology report.

"We'll also find out what treatment plan each doctor recommends next," he says. "From what I've read, I expect they'll suggest radiation and chemotherapy."

Joe expresses concern about the side effects of both options and says he wants to be sure we understand them.

"I don't want to spend the next several months so ill from the treatment that I'm practically an invalid," he says. "Lynn, I want to spend as much time with you and Greg enjoying ourselves. I know that I have a finite amount of time, but I just wish we could understand how much time there might be.

"Let's talk to the doctors about this and then decide," he adds. "Please, I trust these doctors but don't understand what the options may be. I feel better than I did before the surgery and want to continue to get better."

I'm helping Joe get dressed as he talks. He's quite definite about the clothes he wears and the colors he chooses. He likes navy, red, cornflower blue, black, and gray–*never* green or yellow. Maybe pink or turquoise as dress shirts for work. He's practical in what he wears casually. Today he wears a buttoned knit long-sleeved navy top, a navy zip-up windbreaker, and long navy workout pants. I've never seen a man with so many pairs of tennis shoes and walking shoes, and he's wearing his current favorite ones now. I pack the car, and Jane is also ready with her things.

The drive to MGH is the usual craziness, with what seems like an infinite number of semi-trucks all speeding and changing lanes with disregard for cars. We arrive in a little over two hours, and I drive Joe and Jane to the main admitting entrance where I can drop them off. I'm impressed by the volunteers who help Joe out of the car and into a wheelchair. He wants to do some walking while we're here, but he'll start in a chair. Jane stays with Joe while I park the car in the parking garage. Once I join them, walker in tow, we get directions to our first appointment with the radiation oncologist, Dr. O.

We have directions to the Cox Building from the main admittance area, and we proceed past the main lobby desk, past the coffee and donut arena on the right, turn right past the gift shop, past the hair salon (which is a good find), and to a new group of elevators on the right. Next, we go down two floors and exit to our left to a windowless corridor with brown carpet and white walls. The lighting is fluorescent and very artificially bright. The area is practically deserted—a sharp contrast to the bustling, people-jammed hallways we used to get here. Joe checks himself in, and then we wait in a small waiting room where there's only one other person sitting.

I'm out of sorts and tense from the drive to MGH as well as from the unease of navigating to a new place in such a massive hospital complex. Joe is calm, patient, and very kind to the doctor's assistant as she approaches us to move to an office. He wants to get out of his wheelchair and sit in on one of the chairs offered to us, so I leave the wheelchair outside the office. A younger man with dark hair and a beard enters the room and introduces himself as a radiation oncologist. He immediately begins describing the steps of radiation treatment, talking about the imaging process that will be used to create the head mask that Joe will wear during the treatment. He discusses the cutting-edge technology and accuracy of the process as they focus on the radiation sites surrounding the resection Joe had. He tells us Joe will have a total of 30 radiation sessions over six weeks, on a cycle of five days a week followed by two days off. He takes about ten minutes explaining process steps and then asks if we have any questions. We've been following his description closely, and with our technical background in 3D imaging and additive manufacturing, we have no questions for him. We thank him for his time, and he tells us Dr. O will see us shortly.

Dr. O then comes into the room, closes the door behind him, and introduces himself. He apologizes for being late, explaining that he was in another building for a meeting that was longer than planned. He's warm and friendly and smiles a lot. He begins to examine Joe. By now, we're becoming used to the exam. Dr. O checks Joe's eyes motion capability, has him close his eyes and lift each arm separately, and asks him to touch his nose. He checks Joe's arm and leg strength and asks him about his eating and his activity level. He then asks if we have any questions about the radiation treatment. We tell him we don't have questions about radiation but would like to understand other treatment options. Joe is trying to understand how the treatment will make him feel and how it might actually benefit him.

Dr. O explains that the purpose of follow-up treatment for glioma is to prevent reoccurrence of the tumor. The radiation is targeted around the resection boundary with brain tissue and provides further treatment to destroy any cells that could cause regrowth. The radiation path follows the perimeter of the resection site in three dimensions. We ask him about the success rate of the procedure, and he tells us it's based on each individual case. He explains that it can extend a person's life from months to years, depending on the type of tumor, how much of it was removed during the resection, and how responsive it is to radiation. He shows us an image of an MRI that was taken immediately after the surgery and tells us that 99 percent of the tumor was removed, which is considered quite successful. He says that he can't tell us exactly how much it will help but that he believes it will recur more quickly without radiation, although he can't quantify. Joe asks about side effects, and Dr. O explains that the radiation effects are cumulative* and that Joe may experience fatigue over the course of treatment. We inquire about nausea and are told it's not typical. Joe decides to move forward with the procedure, and we ask Dr. O if it's possible to have the mask imaging done while we're in town since we live in Connecticut. He's very obliging and says he'll try to arrange it for us. After Dr. O leaves, Joe comments on how much he liked Dr. O and how he made him feel very comfortable.

After we find out that Joe's appointment for the mask imaging has been set up for tomorrow, we ask for directions to the cafeteria. We proceed precariously through the myriad of busy hallways to yet another building, and I pick out our lunches. Jane asks Joe a few questions while I get our food, and then she gets her own food. I'm afraid to leave Joe alone—it's so busy here that if he goes somewhere, I might have trouble finding him. The cafeteria clientele includes patients, caregivers, doctors, nurses, administrative staff, and cafeteria workers. By the time we finish our lunch, the crowd and noise level have waned. The lunch gives us all a little nourishment, and I feel better afterward.

We next go to the Yawkey Building via a long walk through the main administrative entrance and the Lunder Building. Joe decides he wants to use his walker, so Jane pushes the wheelchair behind him while I walk next to him. It's still very crowded, but not very many people yield to us despite Joe's obvious impairment.

We've been to the 9th floor office area of the Yawkey Building once before, when Joe got his initial diagnosis from Dr. N. Today the waiting room is mostly occupied, and we find a place for Joe to sit while I check him in for his appointment. Fifteen minutes later, Joe is called into the office. Both Jane and I go with him, and we sit in the two extra chairs in the room while Joe sits on the exam table. There's hardly any room for the nurse when she steps into the room.

The nurse, whom I'll call "Nurse S," introduces herself, and Joe immediately introduces Jane and me before he says, "How are things with you today, S?" She smiles and says that she's having a busy day but that things are going well. She explains that she and another nurse are going to determine whether the incision is healed enough for the staples to be removed. While we're waiting, Joe asks her about her background and tells her he's from Tennessee. He jokingly says he learned to wear shoes after he moved to Connecticut. She laughs and asks him about moonshine, so he jokes that he hasn't had his daily dose but hopes to soon.

Soon the other nurse joins her, and they examine the incision and agree to remove the staples. Joe winces occasionally as the staples are removed, and he comments that it stings a little. When the last one is out, Joe says, "Thank goodness all 33 are removed!"

The nurse wipes the incision with alcohol after she says to Joe, "This is going to hurt a little"—which we all know means it's *really* going to hurt. She explains that the incision may start to itch as the incision continues to heal, and she recommends putting a very small amount of petroleum jelly on it if it does. She gives me several small sample tubes to use as needed. We all say goodbye before we leave the patient room.

At the Yawkey reception desk, I request directions to the MGH imaging center for Joe's scheduled MRI. The doctors will compare it to the MRI from before the surgery, and they'll compare it against another MRI after his radiation therapy has been completed. What a surprise—the imaging center is in another building we haven't been to yet.

It's 4:30 p.m., and the hospital is less crowded than it normally is in the middle of the day, although it's not completely quiet. Until now, we had a hospital orderly directing us to the MRI testing area and leading us through corridors not open to the general population. Today, it's another new route through the hospital to discover the patient MRI entrance. I think Christopher Columbus had better tools for navigating than the poor signage we use to find our way around. Eventually we find the MRI test location and Joe is checked in. Because Joe feels claustrophobic when he has an MRI done, I give him the sedative Dr. O prescribed for him. The MRI technician asks Joe to change his clothes and put on a hospital gown, so I wait for him outside the changing room. And wait and wait and wait. Finally, I knock on the changing room door and go in. Joe is sitting on a bench, and he hasn't started to change his clothes.

"What have you been doing in here?" I scold him lightly.

He looks at me, smiles his best smile, and shrugs.

"I decided to sit down for a minute," he responds. "What am I supposed to be doing?"

I'm confused, not understanding what's going on, but I start helping him change. He follows my instructions, but his arms are heavy when we take off his shirt, the left arm heavier than the right. I'm no expert, but I don't think he's had a stroke or a seizure—he seems alert, just very relaxed. Finally, it dawns on me that it must be the medicine prescribed to relax him. Well, it certainly seems to have done the job. I promise myself that I'll cut the pill in half for the next MRI. Once Joe is ready, I ask him to sit in the wheelchair to be rolled to the MRI area. I'm worried that his knees will buckle if he tries to walk. The MRI process takes close to an hour, and I hope the medicine wears off a little by then.

Afterward, Joe is quite jolly as he returns in his wheelchair. He smiles and waves at me, and he jokes with the MRI technician, talking about what it's like undergoing the test. The technician is a little wide-eyed as he tells me Joe can change his clothes and we can leave. It's a little easier to help Joe get dressed than it was before the test, but he's definitely uninhibited. He puts his arm around me while I'm helping him, gives me a kiss, and tells me he loves me. I manage to help him dress and then help him into the wheelchair. He smiles and waves at the receptionist as we leave, telling her to have a great day. As I wheel him to the main entrance, he smiles and talks to everyone we pass, asking them how they're doing or wishing them a good evening.

Joe and Jane wait in the lobby near the exit doors while I get the car from the parking garage. Once again, we have terrific assistance from the volunteers who help patients leaving the hospital. Two young men help Joe into the car, being very careful that he does not hit his head. They won't accept a tip from me, and they wave me off as they push the wheelchair onto the sidewalk.

It's been a long stressful day, and I wonder how Joe had the stamina for everything we did today. He rests with the front seat slightly reclined as I drive to Greg's apartment in Brookline. There's not much talking as I drive through the Boston traffic. It's dark, and we luckily miss some of the rush-hour traffic. Greg meets us in the parking lot of his apartment building and helps Joe with his walker. We coordinated with Greg late this afternoon for dinner plans, so he had food delivered already. Once we're situated in the apartment, we eat our food and fill Greg in on the day's events. Even though Joe is tired, he has renewed energy with Greg. He exaggerates the staple removal process and makes a big deal about *33 staples* being removed. He mimics the process and the sound each staple made when dropped into the plastic container the nurse used. He describes the staple removal tool as "gargantuan pliers, bigger than anything even a dentist would use." A bit of an exaggeration, but it's funny the way he says it.

Shortly after we eat, I help Joe get ready for bed. He still needs to sleep on his back propped up on pillows, so I help arrange them once his clothes are changed. As soon as he leans back on the pillows, he closes his eyes. I sit on the bed next to him until I hear his steady deep breathing. I then go into the living room and blow up the mattress that Jane will sleep on. It's a queen-size mattress, so putting the sheets on is challenging. Jane is rummaging through her suitcase for the things she needs to prepare for bed.

◆

On Thursday morning, we arrive at MGH for Joe's appointment for the 3D scanning to make the mask for his radiation treatment. Once again, we find our way through the busy hospital corridors to the basement of the Cox Building. We're there a couple of hours for the process, which Joe explains to me later.

Joe says they conducted a simulation using CT scans* of the resection site, with barium in his IV for contrast. They had him lie on a padded table, with bolsters supporting his lower back and knees, which helped him feel more comfortable.

After the scans, Joe says, they made the mold by putting some gel and a papier-mâché-like material on his face and head. He tells me that the material was on for about fifteen minutes but that it seemed like forever. He says they showed him a sample finished mask—a mesh-like structure that will be pressed on his forehead, on the sides of his head, and under his chin.

"I'm glad it's over," he says. "My back is stiff from lying on the table for so long. It was so creepy to have the papier-mâché stuff on me, even though I could breathe with no problem."

Joe explains that the doctors will develop a radiation scan plan after the scans are coordinated with the MRI results from yesterday. He's calm, but he tells me he doesn't mind leaving soon. We didn't realize that all these steps would be completed today—we knew about the CT scans but not about the mask being made. When I ask about it as we're leaving, they explain they were trying to help reduce our travel to and from Connecticut, so they arranged for a longer appointment today. We appreciate that, as it was very thoughtful.

We have some time between appointments, so we walk to the cafeteria to buy lunches to go. We then go the 6th floor atrium of the Lunder Building and make a "hospital picnic." We sit in the sun that's shining through the windows of the atrium ceiling and enjoy the warmth, shedding our coats and sweaters while we eat. Our sandwiches are spread on one of the round tables. After Joe finishes eating, he leans back in his chair, closes his eyes, and nods off a little. I check the weather because we're planning to drive home after our appointment at 2 p.m. Uh-oh, the forecast is calling for snow in the early evening. With any luck, we'll be on our way by 3 p.m. and will beat the bad weather.

Joe has alternated using the walker and the wheelchair throughout the day. Now, he uses his walker as we leave the atrium and head over to the 9th floor of the Yawkey Building. We check in, sit down, and wait until about 2:30 p.m. before we're called in to the exam room, which is crowded with Joe, Jane, and me. A nurse who introduces herself as N performs the usual exam that Joe has been getting since his surgery, and she tells us everything looks good. I ask her if the pathology report is available, and she explains that the doctor will discuss it with us when he sees us. It's now 3 p.m.

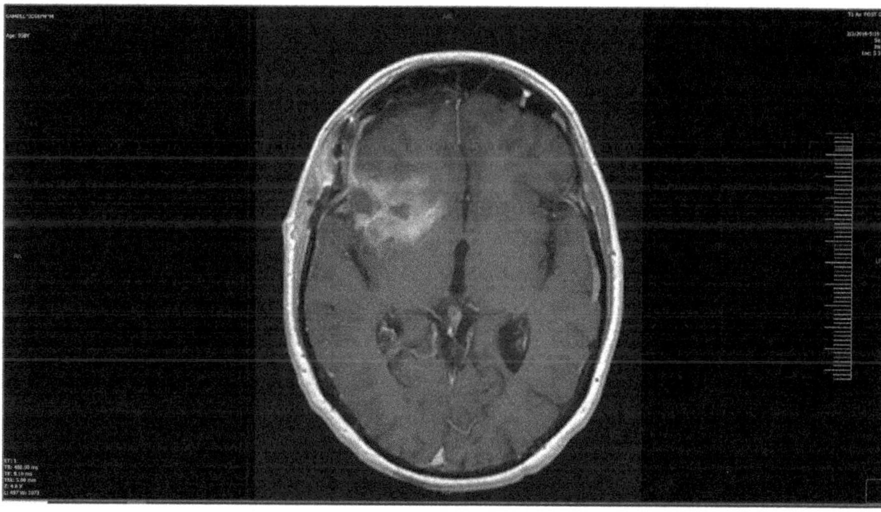

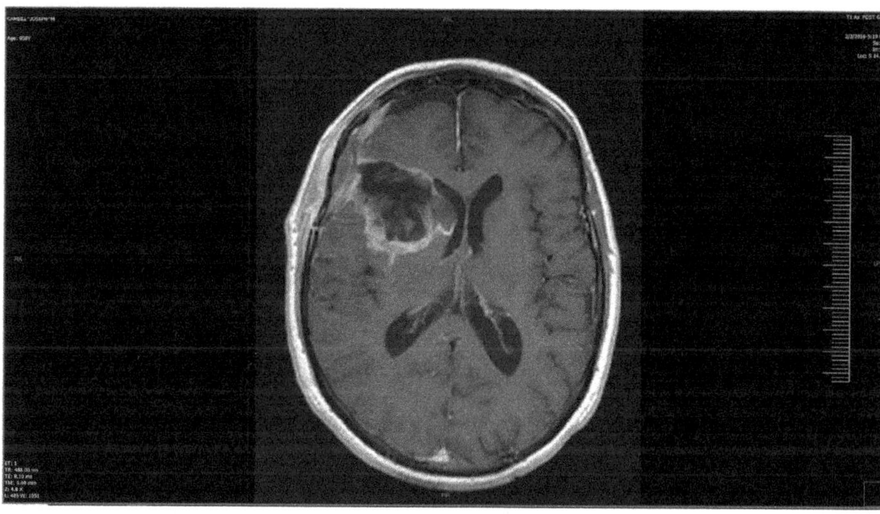

Dr. D, the brain neuro-oncologist, introduces himself when he comes in. It's hard to tell how old he is—maybe mid 40s? He has dark wavy hair, is 5'9" or so, and speaks with what I think is a German accent. He shakes Joe's hand and examines the incision. He completes the now-familiar exam and tells us Joe is doing well. He wants to see Joe walk around in the room and down the aisle unassisted, and Joe does it well. Hah—maybe he doesn't need the walker as much as we both thought.

Dr. D begins discussing proposed treatments. He explains that the tumor pathology shows that Joe's tumor is a glioblastoma multiforme, unmethylated, which is a grade IV astrocytoma. He describes three types of possible treatment plans in conjunction with radiation:

1.Bevacizumab* + lomustine*

2.Bevacizumab + temozolomide*

3.A clinical trial*

I don't understand what he's telling us, and neither does Joe. So we start with our engineer-type questions. What are the benefits of each treatment? Which treatment is most likely to reduce the chance of tumor regrowth and spreading? What is the life expectancy from each of these treatments? What are the side effects and quality of life with each?

It takes some prodding and asking the questions in different ways for us to understand how treatable Joe's glioblastoma is. Unmethylated tumors are more resistant to the first two treatments than methylated tumors, with a success rate of about 20 percent…but it depends on the individual case. *It depends on the individual case*—Joe and I have been hearing that since his diagnosis, and it's so frustrating. Why can't we be given his specific likelihood of success? I ask for a copy of the pathology report while we're discussing treatment options. The report states that the epidermal growth factor receptor (EGFR)* is ">25:1 – too numerous to count." A ratio greater than 5.0 or clustered EGFR signals that are too numerous to count would be considered "highly amplified." I ask what that means, because it sounds scary to the untrained individual like me. Dr. D hesitates before explaining that Joe's tumor is consistent with type 4 glioblastoma, which is aggressive. And fast growing. Factor in unmethylated and it means the tumor is resistant to more-conventional oncology treatments. Okay, now I finally understand it. That's why treatment option 3 was included. In my words, the worst of the worst. My head is pounding as I try to process the news. What do we do now?

I can see that Joe is following my questions and the doctor's answers. He understands what it means. It's not what we hoped for—*not at all.* We then ask questions about the clinical trial. It's a phase 2 clinical trial* of a type of immunotherapy* that can possibly prevent cancer growth by stimulating the immune system. The trial, targeted for unmethylated tumors, involves using an antibody to stimulate the immune system in combination with radiation treatment that causes cell death and release of tumor proteins, which will increase the immune activity of the trial drug. Dr. D concludes the discussion with us and suggests that we think things over and get back to him in a few days. If we decide to participate in the clinical trial, he must apply on our behalf to see if Joe is accepted into the trial. The doctor says the process will take some time, so the sooner we get started, the better.

Okay, now we have more information than we know what to do with. I'm totally slammed from the recent news. Joe looks tired and is sagging a bit. I pick Joe and Jane up at the hospital entry point and start the drive home. It's almost 5 p.m., and we're caught in the traffic leaving Boston. It's already dark and the road is inky black even with the street lights on I-90 W. Traffic is flying by, and then it starts to snow. And does it ever snow. Big heavy flakes, sticking to the car body, the windshield, and the road surface. I'm in the right lane and the traffic is moving slowly, with poor visibility. We drive for about 30 minutes and still haven't reached the first toll booth for I-90 W. Realizing it's only going to get worse, I decide we should find a hotel and stay in Boston for the night. I pull off the interstate and we find a hotel with a restaurant. Joe and I talk about what we learned from Dr. D this afternoon. Joe is already concluding that the clinical trial is his best chance. I'm concerned, feeling like my husband will be a lab rat—an experiment for some company developing a new drug. We discuss the pros and cons and decide to talk more in the morning.

The next morning, we drive to Connecticut in clear weather with the roads free of snow. Joe and I discuss the options on the way home and into the afternoon. Jane asks questions and repeatedly tells Joe that he'll be fine and there's nothing to worry about. She tells us she has friends who've had cancer and lived for more than 20 years after being diagnosed and treated! Of course, not this type of cancer, but hey, who can tell? The decision is ultimately Joe's. He decides he'd like to participate in the clinical trial as the conventional treatments have such a low likelihood of effectiveness. We let Dr. D know our choice and he starts the process of applying for the trial study.

After our recent travel difficulty, Joe and I decide driving to Boston daily for radiation treatment is a bad move. But where will we live for six weeks if we stay in Boston? We can't stay with Greg—he has a roommate. We need to find somewhere near the hospital, because I'm concerned that the back-and-forth to the hospital will be overwhelming as Joe becomes weaker from the radiation. I research hotels near MGH and find out it would be at least $300 a night for a hotel with no kitchen or laundry area. I check for locations farther away and find places that would be 30 to 45 minutes away, but even those are more than $200 a night. What's the point? Way too difficult, also. I talk to Greg about it, and he suggests I look at Airbnb.

I've never used Airbnb before and don't know if it's even a credible option. Greg explains how I can download the app and set up a profile. He says he's used it many times and that it's great. I then start the process and for many days review potential places to stay. I find several, but none are available for the six-week interval we need it for. I finally find a place on Beacon Street—a 300-square-foot one-bedroom, one-bathroom apartment with an efficiency-like kitchen in a high-rise condominium building. It has a laundry room on the same floor, there's a doorman, and it's less than a mile from the hospital. It's $120 a night and is available for the six-week period we need it for—perfect! Greg checks the building out for us and tells us it's in a good location. There are restaurants nearby, with Boston Common and Boston Public Gardens within walking distance.

I arrange for our cats to be taken care of and for our mail to be sent to us in Boston during the six weeks we'll be gone—I need to be sure our bills are paid while we're away. Over the two-week period before we leave for Boston, Joe continues with his physical and occupational therapy. I call his supervisor Chris and explain the situation to him; then I visit my boss and explain face-to-face. I request a longer leave of absence and tell him I probably won't return to work—I want to be with Joe for as long as I can. I understand now that the probability of a successful long-term outcome is unlikely. I have no idea how long we'll be together, but I think five years is a dream. Who knows though—maybe the clinical trial will be a homerun for Joe. I sure hope so.

Jane plans on leaving a few days after we return from MGH. Joe says he'd like to make sure several items that belonged to his parents would be available to her and their brother if they'd like them. He approaches Jane about it, but Jane is understandably upset and won't accept the likely outcome of his illness. She decides she'll take all the items with her to Colorado. It was a difficult afternoon for both Joe and Jane, but I'm glad they discussed it and that the items are with Jane. Greg doesn't want any of them, and neither do I.

I understand that Jane is undeniably shaken knowing she'll be losing her brother sooner rather than later. I also understand that she doesn't know how to help, as none of us know what to do. We have no control over the situation, so the best we can do is make things as easy for Joe as possible. This is the time to think about Joe and what he needs.

Joe and I refuse to give up even though we recognize that the treatment is going to be more challenging than we originally thought. So when Dr. D calls to tell us Joe is accepted into the clinical trial, we're very happy, because Joe believes it's his best chance.

At the end of the two weeks, Joe is walking mostly unassisted. He still needs a little help getting dressed and showering, but he manages reasonably well. His incision has continued to heal and fortunately shows no sign of redness or infection. Preparations have been made for our six-week stay in Boston. The one outstanding concern is where to park my car once we're there, but Greg is working on that. Greg comes to Connecticut the weekend we plan to drive to Boston. On Saturday, I take my car to have snow tires installed because we're expecting a fair amount of snow in February and March. The car is packed Sunday morning, and we're ready to go to Boston!

Chapter 4: Follow-up

False she was, and unrelenting;
When my last joys strewed the ground,
Even Sorrow saw, repenting,
Those sad relics scattered round

Emily Brontë

It's February 15, 2016—Presidents Day—and we're ready to move to Boston temporarily for the next steps in Joe's treatment. Joe made the decision to have radiation treatments and to participate in a clinical immunotherapy infusion* study. He had weighed the choices carefully and vetted each option with MGH doctors and our understanding of the risks versus possible outcome. As we prepare for the drive to Boston, I feel so optimistic about Joe's future and so relieved that decisions have been made. Even though we understand that the pathology report results suggest that the likelihood of treatment success may be low, we believe we've chosen the best possible path forward. Joe appears stronger, is walking with his walker more confidently, and continues to be humorous and hopeful. He accepts that he's still recovering from his surgery, but he knows he's getting better every day. The final preparations for the drive are complete, and we're excited to start this part of Joe's treatment.

Joe rides in the passenger seat, and Greg is crowded in the back seat. I brought Joe's favorite pillows, a shower chair, a walker, nonslip bath and shower mats, a raised toilet seat, bathroom railings, suitcases with winter gear, a laptop computer, a media-streaming player, electrical cords, paper products, cleaning products, and some food. We're ready to hunker down in the Airbnb condominium.

The drive starts out as a typical drive to Boston—that is, until an alert light on my car instrument panel indicates a problem with one of the tires. It has just started to snow lightly, but it's enough to make the roads a little slippery. We're on I-90E near the Sturbridge exit. I pull off the interstate to look for somewhere to have the tire pressure checked and air put in the tires if necessary. Just my luck—I'm having trouble finding one. I feel anxious, responsibility for Joe heavy on my mind. Greg and I use our phones to try to find a tire repair location, finally settling on a place a couple of miles away. Greg's comment to me—"Mom, chill, we'll find something"—only irritates me. I pull in, enter, and ask for someone to look at our tires. Joe, Greg, and I sit in the waiting area for about 30 minutes before someone finally looks at the car. Thankfully, the tires are okay; the tire pressure wasn't reset in the car when the snow tires were installed on Saturday.

It stopped snowing while we were waiting, but the sidewalk and parking lot are an ice slick. We carefully pile back into the car to continue to Boston. Joe and Greg accept the event with ease, joking about the "side trip" and the "fire-breathing dragon" who's navigating. I, on the other hand, am anything but at ease, but at least I can laugh at their descriptions.

Aaah, a new experience, driving through the many one-way streets surrounding the Boston State Capitol area, eventually finding the way to Beacon Street. It starts to snow and is bleak and dreary, with gray skies. There are a couple of bare trees with dark gray-brown limbs, the sidewalk surrounding their roots. I see a parking lot next to the apartment building and am happy something is so close to where we'll be staying. I turn left into the lot and am immediately greeted by a man who requests I pay $40 an hour to unload the car. Welcome to the city of exorbitant parking costs.

I try to negotiate a lower price, but he's unrelenting—that is, until he sees Joe getting out of the passenger seat and notices the long, still-pink incision on the side of his head. He looks at me, and in his heavy eastern European accent, he asks me if we're here for medical treatment. My eyes start to fill up with tears; I'm not trying to be manipulative, it just happens. I nod my head and explain that I don't know where to park a car in the city. He strokes his chin with his right hand as he looks down at his feet. He then makes eye contact with me and says he will let me park for a few hours for the $40 rate while we unload. He tells me where a couple of car garages are in the area that I might try after we unload and are settled in. I thank him profusely and move the car deeper into the lot while Greg helps Joe use his walker and navigate into the building.

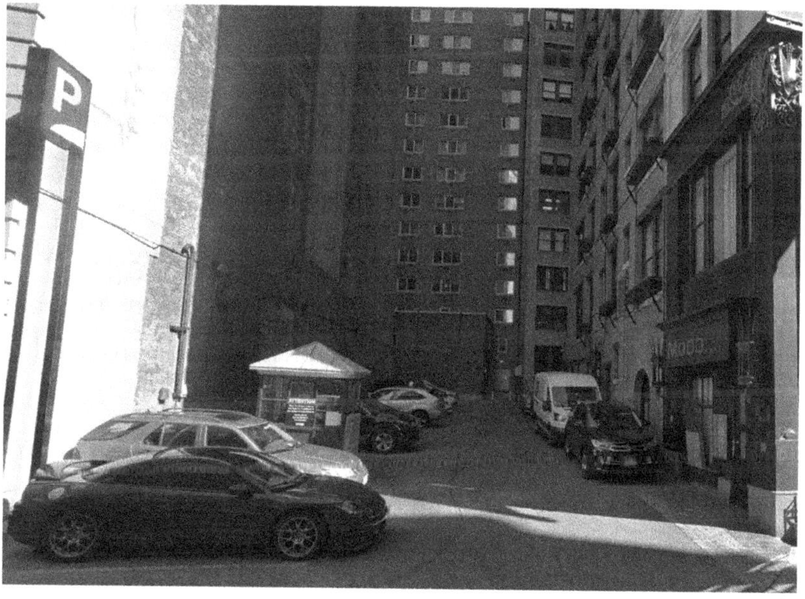

I've never used Airbnb before, and I imagine the many ways that things can go awry. The rented apartment is actually in a condominium building with few short-term rentals. When I was looking for a place to stay, one requirement was that it have no or very few steps leading into the building. With Joe's walking capability and the winter weather, we need to minimize risk of falling. I approach the front entryway and am excited to see that there are no steps, as advertised. I enter the first-floor lobby, walk to the concierge desk, and explain that I'm picking up a key for 11B. The concierge isn't very friendly as he hands me a legal-size manila envelope. I can feel a key through the paper and nod to Joe and Greg to proceed to the elevators on our right.

The lobby is old but very clean. It has ornate columns and cream marble floors inlaid with black corner decorative marble. A small settee sofa and two armchairs are positioned near the far wall of the lobby. We have the elevator to ourselves as we rise to the 11th floor. As we exit the elevator, we see the gold dome of the State House through the windows straight ahead. It's quite postcard picturesque, and we stop to admire the view. We can also see a little of the Boston Commons park. We turn left and walk to the end of the hall, and our rented condominium is immediately on our left. A set of stairs to the left of our doorway appears to go down, perhaps to the lobby. I'll decide to check it out later.

The key is a bit tricky to engage, but I figure out that the door will open if I pull the door toward me as I turn the key. We enter a small living area with a blue microfiber sofa, two chairs, a 36" round dinette with three chairs and a three-foot-high open-shelf, dark-brown cabinet with a small TV on the top shelf. Directly across from the door are two windows with a radiator below the windows. The condominium is a corner unit, so we have a nice view of the buildings on Beacon Street.

So far, it looks exactly like the Airbnb photos. A counter-height wall separates the living room from a very compact but fully equipped galley-style kitchen with a pass-through to the living area. The refrigerator is quite small, but there's a microwave and a kitchen range with an oven. The kitchen area will be functional, but there's room for only one person at a time in the tiny area. A short hallway separates the living room from the bedroom, which is also minimal—a queen-size bed and an end table are all there's room for. But at least there are several closets, which will give us room for our clothes. The bathroom, however, is a bit of a problem. It has a tub and shower, which means Joe will need to step over the tub to take a shower. I'm so glad I brought the nonslip shower pad and floor rugs. As soon as Joe sees the bathroom, he jokes that it's as small as an airplane bathroom—which isn't much of an exaggeration.

Joe rests while Greg and I make several trips to the car to bring our things up to the condominium. On the last trip, the parking lot attendant waves me over and tells me I need to move my car. Greg and I decide that Greg will drive my car to his apartment building in Brookline where he can park the car in a visitor parking spot, then take a ride-sharing service back to Beacon Street. I take the last suitcase up to the condominium and join Joe sitting on the sofa. As I look around the condominium, I realize it will be manageable even though it's very tiny. I hate the simulated oak laminate flooring and the worn look of the dinged baseboards and doors. It isn't that anything is particularly dirty, but it looks very used. The window blinds are cheap plastic verticals that feel flimsy when I adjust them. The owner left us a packet of information on the table explaining how to use the TV and telling us we may need to open the windows to cool the condominium occasionally because the heating is very efficient in our unit. I find the media-streaming device and connect it to the TV. It takes a few tries to get it to work, but finally we have all the TV stations we'd have at our home in Connecticut. Joe and I have some adjusting to do to live in this small area. We both rest a little as we wait for Greg to return.

By the time Greg returns, Joe and I both had sandwiches and are feeling refreshed and I put our clothes, food, and cleaning supplies away. I hope I can remember where I put things, but at least there won't be many places to search if I can't find them right away. I need to go to a grocery store to pick up all the things we'll need over the next few days, so I use my phone to find the closest one. There's a Whole Foods about a mile away. Now that doesn't sound too far, does it?

I can't say I'm known for finding my way around, even with a navigation system. Somehow, I manage to complicate directions, second guessing what they really mean. I know that finding the grocery store will be tricky for me in an area I'm not familiar with. As I look out the window, I see it's snowing again. Greg downloads a navigation system to my phone and routes the path to the Whole Foods store for me. He's a millennial, and he lives off apps. I would send him to the store for me, but I need to know how to do this myself. There'll be many times over the next few weeks when I'll need to go and get groceries. Besides, Greg would probably bring back things that I wouldn't pick out and I'd have to improvise with recipes. I'm not very adept at that, either.

Joe and Greg look comfortable as I bundle up with coat, hat, scarf, and gloves for the walk to the store. I don't mind a small adventure; in fact, I look forward to it a little. I'm unfamiliar with my surroundings as I leave the condominium and navigate through the building lobby. I try to make eye contact with the concierge, but he won't acknowledge me. I guess this is the big city way and it isn't very welcoming. I exit the building and turn right on Beacon Street. It's about 3:30 p.m., and the wind is blustering around me. Sunset today will be between 4:30 and 5 p.m. I'd like to be back before dark, but I know I probably won't be. I turn left on Somerset Street, turn left again on Ashton Place, right on Bowdoin Street, and left on Cambridge Street to Whole Foods. The roads are steep and hilly, and several are brick and a little slippery. I'm not visualizing how I got to the store, but I follow the directions successfully.

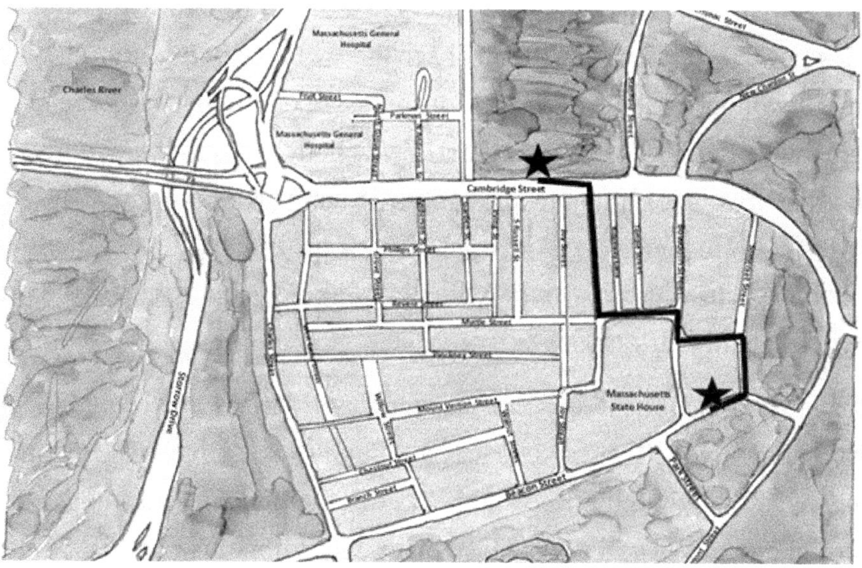

It's close to the end of the day on a Monday, so the store is crowded. It takes longer to find what I came for, because I don't know the store layout. I finally have everything I need, and of course I have a lot to carry back to the condominium. I start the return trip using the navigation system. It tells me to take Cambridge to Bowdoin, but it doesn't have me turn on Ashton Place. What's going on? So in my infinite wisdom, I turn on Ashton, trying to retrace my steps. Big mistake. Before I know it, I'm lost, unable to find Beacon Street. I'm disoriented, frustrated, and cold, and the bags of groceries seem to be getting heavier by the minute. I call Greg on his phone for help navigating, and he tries to direct me but quickly gets annoyed with me as I try to describe where I am. I eventually find my way back, but I don't feel confident about being able to find my way back to the store again. At least I got the food we need for the next few days, even if my confidence is shaken.

When I finally get back to our temporary new home, Joe and Greg are sitting on the couch and in a chair, respectively, and I immediately sense how relaxed and cozy they are. It's a tiny, crowded living area, but somehow it doesn't matter as I see the two men in my life. They have a wonderful father-son relationship built on mutual respect, camaraderie, and sense of humor. They're both very pithy and witty, and they love to exaggerate and imitate situations. Greg is great at parroting a Boston accent and interchanges his usual accent with a Boston accent whimsically. Now they're talking about football and the New England Patriots.

For Joe and me, I heat up some lasagna that I'd made and brought from home, while Greg orders a Thai dinner to be delivered. Greg is a vegan, and the food that Joe and I eat doesn't align with his chosen current culinary restrictions. Once everyone's dinner is ready, we sit together at the dinette and eat. I so love that we're all together, although the circumstances are definitely not what any of us would prefer. After dinner, Greg takes a ride-sharing service to his apartment. He plans to see us again on Thursday after work.

With Greg gone, Joe and I are alone in this new place. The lighting is minimal, and the room is dim and shadowy. Good for watching TV, but not so good for keeping an eye on Joe. His night owl habits haven't returned since his illness, and he now sleeps more than he used to. Typically, he's ready to go to bed at around 9 p.m., and he wakes up at 8 or 9 a.m. unless I roust him earlier. He used to stay up until at least 11 p.m. and get up at around 6:30 a.m. During the winter months, when golf wasn't an option, he'd usually work a lot more, either at the office or from home. He doesn't have many indoor hobbies, unless putting golf balls on an indoor practice mat counts. He likes to read, do an occasional crossword puzzle, and watch TV. Now with work not part of his daily routine, he's spending time on his phone, texting, reading a little, and watching TV. He works around his new medical schedule, which has been very busy. He isn't asking to do more and isn't indicating that he's bored. It's been a month since his surgery, and he appears to be mostly himself except for short term-memory of appointments, taking his pills on time, and understanding how long things take. His sense of time is a bit off.

As we watch TV, I wonder what he's thinking about and whether he notices any change. He's never been a person to talk directly about his feelings. Instead, he uses humor to express what he thinks and feels—not in a biting way, but in a roundabout, sideways type of communication. For example, he'll say something like, "We would've understood the show better if we'd seen all of it" instead of a direct confrontation like, "Why were you late?" Communication is softer, yet the meaning is understood: we would've seen all of the show if I hadn't been late. Asking Joe how he feels or if he notices a change is tricky.

I ask him, "What time are we leaving for the hospital tomorrow?"

"Whatever time you tell me to go," he replies.

We've already discussed the timing several times today: we're leaving at 7:30 a.m. "Yes, but what time are we leaving here?" I ask.

He winks at me and says, "Sometime tomorrow."

I sigh, not sure whether he's joking with me or doesn't remember. So I ask him, "What time do you want to wake up tomorrow so we'll be on time for your appointment?"

He says, "What time do you think I should wake up? Just tell me the time and I'll get up and get ready."

"Joe, do you remember when your appointment is?" I ask.

"Of course I remember—it's tomorrow!" he exclaims.

"Yes, but what time?" I persist.

He gives me a little smile and a shoulder shrug. I know he doesn't remember, so I go over the plan with him again. Joe responds by telling me he's tired and wants to go to sleep.

Our first night trying to sleep in the condominium takes some getting used to. The bed is a queen size instead of a king size like at home. The mattress is supportive enough, but it dips toward the middle a bit. The furnace ticks repeatedly all night long as it struggles to keep up with the temperature setting, since there's no thermostat in the room. We hear the voices of patrons and vendors of nearby Beacon Street bars and restaurants throughout the night from the street below us.

As I rest next to Joe, I ask him how he feels about starting new procedures this week.

He answers, "I don't expect them to be as bad as sticking a needle in my eye."

Well, that really tells me how he feels about it.

◆

At 6:45 a.m. on Tuesday morning, we're in the lobby of the condominium building—me perched on a restuffed firm tan couch and

Joe sitting in one of the armchairs. For the first time, I'm trying to use the ride-sharing app Greg downloaded on my phone so I can request a ride to the hospital. I enter our destination and current location. I get a response that shows a driver is four minutes away and tells us the car's color, make, model, and license plate number. I'm apprehensive about using the service, unsure what it will be like. We exit the building, past the concierge who won't look at us. Joe won't stand for this, so he says "Good Morning" anyway. There's no response from the concierge. We approach the curb and wait there, with Joe using his walker.

Finally, Joe sees a set of headlights flash on and off across the street, and an SUV approaches. The driver gets out of the car, helps Joe get in, and puts his walker in the hatchway. He proceeds to MGH—it's only 1.2 miles away, but it takes us 25 minutes to get there. The driver chats along the way, talking about Boston and sites we can see. He has no difficulty navigating the traffic, and the ride is pleasant enough.

Today Joe is having the fit of his radiation mask checked. The appointment is below ground on the 2nd floor of the Cox Building, and we try to find it without asking for directions. As usual, the hospital is busy and the hallways are crowded. We take at least one wrong turn and have to retrace our steps, so we get to the appointment a little bit late. Joe doesn't want to use a wheelchair this morning, so he's using his walker.

After Joe is checked in, a technician escorts him to the room where the creation of the original mask began. Another tech asks Joe to lie on his back on a flat table, his lower back and knees supported by molded bolsters. The techs adjust the mask on his head and bolt the mask to the table. The mask reminds me of a hockey mask except that it's made from a plastic mesh-like material. It's too tight around the throat and presses too much into his forehead, so they remove the mask and make adjustments until they find an optimum fit. The process takes an hour or so.

Once the process is complete, we're given Joe's radiation schedule for the first week. His sessions will be at 6 p.m. Wednesday through Friday. Next we meet with Dr. O to talk more about the radiation process. Dr. O says each session will take about 45 minutes and will be painless. The radiation scan plan can be completed today, now that the mask has been fitted. He then performs the usual exam, checking Joe's eyes, reflexes, balance, and strength in the left versus right side. He notes that the left side is improved but is slightly weaker than the right, so he recommends that Joe continue physical and occupational therapy while he's at MGH and requests that his office submit the requirement to our insurance company.

Joe has a good rapport with Dr. O and finds it easy to ask him questions. Dr. O explains that Joe's next MRI will be after all radiation sessions are complete, as there can be slight brain variation with the radiation that may influence the results of the MRI. We ask Dr. O a lot of questions about what to expect over the next couple of months, and he reminds us that Joe may feel some fatigue as the radiation process continues because the effects of the radiation are cumulative.* He also explains that there's a small chance they'll use radiation treatment if Joe's glioma regrows. He says the next step will be 3D conformal radiation,* which will follow the perimeter of the tumor resection to help prevent regrowth of the tumor. If the tumor does regrow, though, surgery could be an option depending on the specific location of the tumor.

We ask him how long it typically takes a tumor to regrow, and he smiles a little and jokes about us being engineers. He explains that medicine is not an exact science and is much different from our careers, meaning that every patient is different and that whatever happens in Joe's case will be unique. We tell him about the timelines we've been reading about on the Internet. "Don't believe everything you read on the Internet," he laughs in response.*

When I ask what we should look for that might indicate that something has changed, he tells us that a repeat of his prior symptoms, a seizure, and behavior changes are common signs. Once again, our quest for specific answers turns out to be frustrating. We still don't know how much quality time Joe has, but we do know that a change such as a seizure would be significant.

We have some time before our next appointment, which is with Dr. D. We learn from Dr. O's receptionist that there's another cafeteria in the Cox Building, although it's smaller than the one in the main building. The Cox cafeteria has fewer menu items, but at least it's less crowded than the main cafeteria. We then make our way to the 9th floor of the Yawkey Building.

The admitting desk for Dr. D's office divides two patient waiting areas. Behind the admitting desk is a pass-through hall that opens to each patient waiting area and includes several individual chairs for taking blood, scales for measuring height and weight, and moveable stands for checking blood pressure. The check-in process is disorganized today, and the admitting staff search through many folders before they finally find Joe's.

After Joe is registered and a wristband is attached to his arm, we sit in two of the reclining chairs in the patient waiting room. A very young woman calls Joe's name and we let her know where we're sitting. The woman asks us to follow her through the single door to the doctors' offices. We're sitting in a patient room that looks like all the others we've been in when the door opens and we're introduced to "N." N is a registered nurse who'll be working with Joe while he's in the clinical study. She reviews with Joe a document that describes the clinical study, the risks, possible side effects, the study schedule, and the duration of the study phase. The study will be conducted in conjunction with radiation therapy. After reviewing the document, Joe signs a consent form. His first scheduled treatment is at 10 a.m. tomorrow. He'll have another treatment every two weeks, assuming all goes well.

We leave the appointment at around 3:30 p.m. and walk to the waiting area of the main hospital entrance, where I use the ride-sharing app to take us back to Beacon Street. We wait about fifteen minutes to be picked up, and the drive takes a little longer because of all the traffic near the Capitol area and the Boston Commons park. We're dropped curbside and make our way into the main lobby, a slow but progressive approach. We have difficulty entering the main lobby doors as the concierge will not electronically activate the doors for us. The doors are very heavy for me to maneuver manually, but finally I manage. I've had enough of him and shoot him dagger eyes, but Joe simply smiles at him and wishes him a good afternoon. You catch more bees with honey, of course.

Joe managed the entire day with his walker, not requesting a wheelchair. It's great progress, even though he's tired when we arrive in our condominium. We have a quiet evening, talking about the appointments and comparing our observations over dinner. We both feel very confident in the treatment choices and that we're getting the best care possible at MGH, though we struggle with the unknowns of the treatment benefits. We so wish we had access to more definitive information for Joe's specific evaluation, but we're optimistic that the treatment will delay regrowth of tumors for several years.

◆

On Wednesday, we follow the same routine: shower, breakfast, rideshare to MGH. We arrive close to 10 a.m. for Joe's first infusion treatment in the Yawkey Building. It's a two-step process: we go to Dr. D's office area on the 9th floor of the Yawkey Building for a baseline blood test, then to the infusion center on the 8th floor. We wait an hour or so between the two steps while the blood test results are reviewed. Neither of us has ever been to an infusion center. The waiting room is like other waiting areas we've been to—but it's a very different story once we're called in to the infusion center. There are several private rooms, each with patient seating or a bed and equipped with TV monitors and computers. There are many individual reclining chairs lined up along the sides of hallways, with overhead drapes that can be used to separate the seating areas. Each seating area has a small TV on a low table, a rolling stand for an IV, and a computer monitor. Some of the chairs have a spectacular view of the Charles River, with the water sparkling and sailboats anchored or moving slowly along the river.

Once in the infusion center, Joe is weighed and then is brought to a private room with a reclining bed. We wait for almost two hours, and it's almost lunchtime. Then there's a knock on the door and an elderly woman pushes a rolling three-tier table into our room. On each shelf are sandwiches, drinks, ice cream, and condiments. So we eat lunch while we wait, impatient for the process to begin. Finally, our infusion nurse arrives with a fluid bag that she connects to the IV. She tells us that Joe's vital signs will be taken every fifteen minutes during the infusion and that the infusion will be stopped if anything is irregular. The infusion itself will take two hours, after which Joe will be observed for adverse reactions* or any other problems, she says. Neither of us knew this would be the procedure, so we're learning as we go. I had no idea the entire infusion process would take close to four hours from beginning to end. The nurse explains that the MGH pharmacy mixes Joe's infusion medicine based on the clinical study formula and his exact weight. At each visit, the infusion medicine will be mixed before the infusion starts. When the pharmacy is busy—which it usually is—it takes at least two hours to mix the infusion, the nurse says.

The infusion process begins, and the nurse checks Joe's vital signs repeatedly. Fortunately, there are no problems with his vital signs, and he experiences no adverse reactions. Inwardly, I'm so relieved, as I didn't know how his system would react. He showed no outward sign of being worried during the process, but I find it hard to believe he wasn't.

Joe is observed for an hour after the infusion, still with no unusual reaction. I feel like I've been holding my breath for hours. It's now 3 p.m., and Joe's first radiation session is at 6 p.m. We decide to try to go back and forth to the condominium so Joe can have some downtime between appointments. We ride-share to the condo and have a couple of hours to rest in the quiet yet comfortable tiny living space.

Back to the hospital after a short rest we go, ride-sharing again. It's around 5:15 p.m., and it's much harder to find a ride-share driver than in the morning. Several drivers respond but then cancel, and I'm worried we'll be late for the first radiation treatment. Finally, a driver shows up and we're on our way to MGH. Once we arrive, Joe decides to use a wheelchair, so I push the chair while he balances the walker on the footrests of the chair. We manage to make it work, and once again we're going to a place in the hospital we've never been. This time we're going to the Lunder Building, but down three floors. The elevator is readily accessible this time of day, now 5:45 p.m.

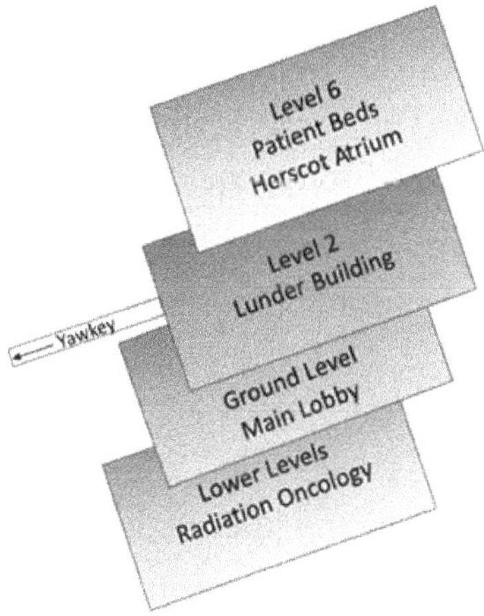

Lunder Building

When we exit the elevator, in front of us is a small reception area with a desk facing the elevator. Fortunately there's someone sitting at the desk, so we proceed to check Joe in. Joe is given a card that provides access to the radiation treatment area and we're shown the way to the radiation location. When the double wood entryway doors open, we're taken to a computer on our right. We're told we should scan the card to electronically alert the radiation technicians that we're here. We take a seat in the waiting area, which isn't very large for a hospital the size of MGH. There are close to 20 seats of various styles. A few are recliners, one is a massaging recliner, and the remainder are upright upholstered chairs. The area is clean and appears relatively new. Joe is seated in one of the recliners, and I sit opposite him in a standard upholstered chair. We don't wait more than ten minutes before a young man in a white lab gown calls Joe's name. When Joe answers, the technician introduces himself. It's been a long day for Joe, but you wouldn't know it from the polite and smiling response he gives the tech. I hear Joe asking him about his favorite sports as they walk down a hallway to the right. I wait about 45 minutes in the waiting area until Joe and the technician return. I can see a waffle pattern imprint on Joe's forehead as he walks toward me; I presume the imprint is from the radiation mask. Joe shakes hands with the technician and thanks him for his help before asking me for his coat. We go through the logistics of finding the main lobby, summoning a ride-share car, and riding to the condo, and we arrive by around 7:30 p.m.

Once we're settled in to our home away from home, Joe explains the radiation treatment process. He said that once he was lying down on the padded table with his back and knees supported, the techs strapped him down across his chest and legs, positioned the mask on his face, and bolted the mask to the table. The techs were very considerate, adjusting the back support several times until he was comfortable and playing his choice of music to make the process as tolerable as possible, he says.

Via computer, the techs move the table and the radiation equipment throughout the process to target different locations with the radiation. The mask was tight and the feeling of being unable to move made him very uncomfortable, but he was careful to stay still because the techs told him it could cause the radiation to miss its target. He tells me he was relieved when the mask was unbolted and removed.

"I tried to focus on the music and think about how the process is helping me," he says. "Now that I know what to expect, I can do it."

Joe just describes the process in a steady, matter-of-fact tone. No particular emotion, no "Why me, this is so hard"—just the facts, ma'am. I let him explain, and I listen to him without asking him any questions. I hope that giving him a chance to talk about the process will help him. After dinner, he goes to bed and is asleep minutes after he rests his head on the pillow.

I sit in the living room, thinking about the day's events. I'm tired myself, and I'm not even the patient who had an infusion and radiation treatment! I can't believe how Joe has so much physical and emotional strength. He didn't complain once throughout the day. And I know the infusion must've hurt. An IV was in his arm for several hours—having that inserted and removed is painful! Also, I could tell that the radiation process was difficult for him. His back must've hurt, lying in one position for so long and having his head and neck totally fixed in place. How did he stand it? I have my rosary with me, and I pray for Joe to recover from this disease.

For as long as I've known Joe, he's had a way of making me and everyone else he meets feel like they're special to him. I've studied how he does this over the years, but I still don't know how he does it. He makes direct eye contact with whomever he's talking to, he smiles a lot, and he looks for something about each person he meets that he can connect with. Then he uses humor in situations that he shares with the person and exaggerates what's happening. I know it's what he does. But there's more to this: it comes with a generosity of spirit from Joe trying to connect with you and have fun with you. I've known for many, many years how lucky I am to have Joe in my life. There are people who take from life and there are those who give to life. I've always known Joe to be one of the givers.

I think about what we'd be doing if we were in Connecticut and Joe wasn't sick. The golf season is approaching, starting in April. Joe would be beginning to prepare for it. He has a kind of ritual he goes through each year. I smile when I remember what it is, and I shake my head as I think about parts of his routine: first, he finds his favorite golf shoes and cleans them—sometimes in the garage and sometimes outside, because I've forbidden him from cleaning them in the house.

Then he replaces any cleats that need repair. He takes everything out of his golf bag and brings it into the house. I always hate that, because inevitably, there's so much junk that accumulated in the various pockets of his golf bag and he spreads it all out on the dining room table to inspect. There are golf balls, tees, markers, old scorecards, golf hats, sunscreen, insect repellent, raingear, miscellaneous receipts from who knows where, socks, loose change, and I'm sure much more. How did all this stuff fit in one golf bag?

Joe takes the boxes that the golf balls come in and separates the lids from the bottoms. Then he fills the boxes with the various items, sorted by category. Once that's finished, he selects his favorite items and puts them back into his golf bag. Then he stores the rest of the items in the garage for "later" in the season. He has several of these boxes already stored, and they never seem to find their way out of the garage once he has sorted them and saved them for "later." He then inspects his golf clubs and starts cleaning them in the kitchen sink. (Oh, I really love this part of the process.) Then he studies the club grips and, if necessary, puts them aside to be regripped for the season. It usually takes the better part of a day. Then, over the next week or so, Joe will assess his golf wardrobe and organize his closet by color so he can quickly select a golf shirt. He's always organized and ready to play when the season starts. But now, he hasn't mentioned golf once since his surgery.

◆

On Thursday morning, Joe sleeps in until around 9:30 a.m. I log in to my work computer and continue with various tasks, mostly focusing on email correspondence. While Joe is eating breakfast, my cell phone rings. It's a physical therapist from MGH, asking to schedule Joe for an evaluation. She has an opening for 1 p.m. today, so we agree to meet with her later.

I do some laundry in the morning in a common laundry room on the 11th floor. The apartment is so tiny that there's nowhere to put worn clothing, so I need to keep up with laundry regularly. Joe focuses on his phone, reading various news reports and texting his colleagues at work. We talk about work, comparing what each of us knows about what's going on. Some personnel changes are being made with senior management, and we're interested in what's happening.

Before we know it, it's time to leave for the hospital. Once again, we ride-share from the lobby and have pretty good luck finding a driver. The drive is becoming somewhat routine for us. When we walk in through the main entryway, we find that the physical therapy area is to the right of the main lobby on the 1st floor. Joe uses his walker as we carefully proceed along a long corridor, turning right halfway down into the waiting room of the physical therapy reception area. I check Joe in while he sits down, and then we wait for fifteen minutes or so. Everywhere we go—whether it's an appointment, a test, or a treatment—we usually wait. It's very rare that we're called into a scheduled visit on time.

When Joe is called, we both go into a physical therapy room. The room is rectangular, maybe 75 yards long by 45 yards wide. Along the wall opposite the entry doors, there are patient beds separated by cloth curtains hanging on ellipse-shaped rails. Most of the curtains are open, and I can see several patients working with therapists. The beds appear to be adjustable, and patients are doing exercises in various positions. I estimate that there are around ten beds. In the middle of the room, near the end lengths, are sets of adjustable parallel bars. Also mounted to the ceiling are straps that patients can use to support their waist or chest when they try to walk.

Joe is introduced to his physical therapist ("M"), who walks with him and asks him to sit on one of the beds. The bed is in the flat position, so M adjusts the height to his leg length. She has a questionnaire and asks him about his health and his current activity level. While he's seated, she has him lift each leg individually and presses down to assess the strength of his legs. She does the same with his arms and then asks him to reach up—first with each arm separately and then with both arms together. She has him stand up and sit down several times, and then she asks him to walk the length of the room with the walker while she stays by his side. Next, she asks him to turn his head to the left and to the right while he walks, and she watches to see if he can walk in a straight line. Lastly, she puts a support belt around his waist and holds it as he walks without the walker. Joe really concentrates and gives his best effort to complete every one of the activities, and he's very tired when he's finally finished. The evaluation takes close to 45 minutes.

M reviews her conclusions with us. She explains that Joe's left side continues to be weaker than his right and he has difficulty walking in a straight line when he turns his head, so she'd like him to work on building his strength and balance. She says she'd like Joe to walk for 20 to 30 minutes every day—twice if he can—and gives us about eight exercises for him to do at least once daily. Some of the exercises are similar to those Joe was doing at home, but they all focus on the same key areas. Some are leg and arm extensions, balance activities, leg lifts, sitting and standing repetitively, and leg bridges. If we can find some stairs, he'll need to practice walking up a couple of stairs and then walk down backwards. M schedules appointments to see Joe twice a week.

It's interesting to me how Joe demonstrates his capability with M, yet doing exercises at home is such a chore for him. He shows a lot of enthusiasm, and I see that visits with her can be motivation for his upcoming home workouts and plan to use this to help him rebuild his skills. She's very pretty, with long chestnut hair and blue eyes, and is strong and athletic looking. She has a patient, easygoing personality. Our physical therapist in Connecticut was quite good, but MGH is a step up. We ride-share back to the apartment so Joe can rest a little before his scheduled radiation appointment.

The radiation treatment is similar to the first one, except this time we know what to expect. There are plenty of seats available in the waiting room, and Joe's appointment starts on time. Yeah!!! Afterward, as Joe approaches me to leave the treatment area, I notice he's joking with the technician about music choices. We ride-share back to the apartment and are home by 7:30 p.m. Tonight, Greg is visiting us. He takes the T from St. James Avenue to the Boston Commons exit and walks to our apartment from there. He calls me from the lobby and asks me to speak to the concierge to let him come upstairs. I request that Greg be put on a list so he can come and go as he likes, but the concierge tells me I'll need to go to the lobby and fill out a form. Okay, so I go to the lobby and fill out the form, and Greg rides the elevator with me to see his dad.

There's no such thing as a silver lining to Joe having this dreadful illness. We made the best treatment choices we knew how to make and decided that MGH was the best option for him. Because MGH is in Boston where Greg lives, we knew we'd be able to see Greg much more frequently than if Joe were treated elsewhere. The three of us are very close, and being together often during this time is a powerful motivator for Joe and me. We're in an unfamiliar place, but once we're together, it quickly becomes a new family setting. Having the three of us together helps Joe and me feel optimistic.

When Greg joins us after work, we eat together, sharing the apartment dinette table and chairs. He's such a breath of fresh air to us after we spent our day in the hospital. He tells us stories about his work, friends, exercise routine, dating (though not much on this subject), and travel plans. We don't talk much about our day, as we want our precious time together to be uplifting for everyone. I still haven't found a permanent solution to parking my car in the city—but to my surprise, Greg tells us over dinner that he has! The property maintenance manager where he rents his apartment has a parking lot across the street from the apartment complex. He agreed to rent us a parking spot for $300 for the six weeks we're in Boston. It turns out that Greg told him about our situation, so he reduced his usual rental price to help us out. I can hardly believe it, and I quickly write a check for Greg to give him before he changes his mind. What an unexpected act of kindness from a person we haven't even met. In my heart, I thank him, and I ask Greg to thank him for us. First the parking attendant next door and now this.

Friday mid morning, Joe decides he wants to go for a walk. We're fortunate that we're very close to the Boston Commons park. Even with the dauntingly cold temperature and the trees and shrubs typical New England brown, gray, and tan, a walk in the park is appealing to both of us. Well, I should say, our first walk was *no* walk in the park.

As we leave our building, Joe is using his walker. We don't know the traffic routine in this area and there are many trucks making deliveries, parking along the curbs of the streets. The sidewalk is uneven, which makes using the walker a bit precarious. We cross Beacon Street and turn right, approaching Park Street. Up and down curbs we go, crossing Park Street while still on Beacon street. On our left is a set of stairs going down to the park, and on our right is the Massachusetts State House. Uh-oh—stairs, and lots of them. Of course Joe can't use a walker on the stairs, so he decides to hold on to the sturdy handrails because he wants to continue to walk a little. I don't like the idea one bit, but I fold the walker up and carry it in one hand and hold Joe's belt in the other as we walk down the stairs slowly, one step at a time. He puts one foot on a stair, then catches up with the other foot on the same stair. We make our way to the end of the stairs, turn right, and walk a short distance to sit on a park bench.

It isn't a particularly pretty day in February—overcast and in the 30s—but we're dressed for the weather and it's a beautiful day to us. Joe managed to get to the park, and more importantly, he *wanted* to. This is our first activity in Boston not associated with a hospital trip, and it's exhilarating to both of us. As we sit on the park bench, we people watch and speculate about where each person may be going. Some people are dressed for work, and we try to guess what their careers might be. Others are clearly enjoying leisure time, so we discuss what we think they do all day. There are a few birds in the park, which are fun to watch as well. Wow, we really sound like older people, don't we? We laugh about this a little and Joe decides we should go back to the apartment. It's slower going back than coming as Joe walks up the set of stairs. But he's very careful, and we pay attention to cars, pedestrians, and delivery workers as we make our way to the condominium.

Every time we enter and leave the building, Joe greets the lobby concierge—always at least a "good morning" and sometimes a "hello,

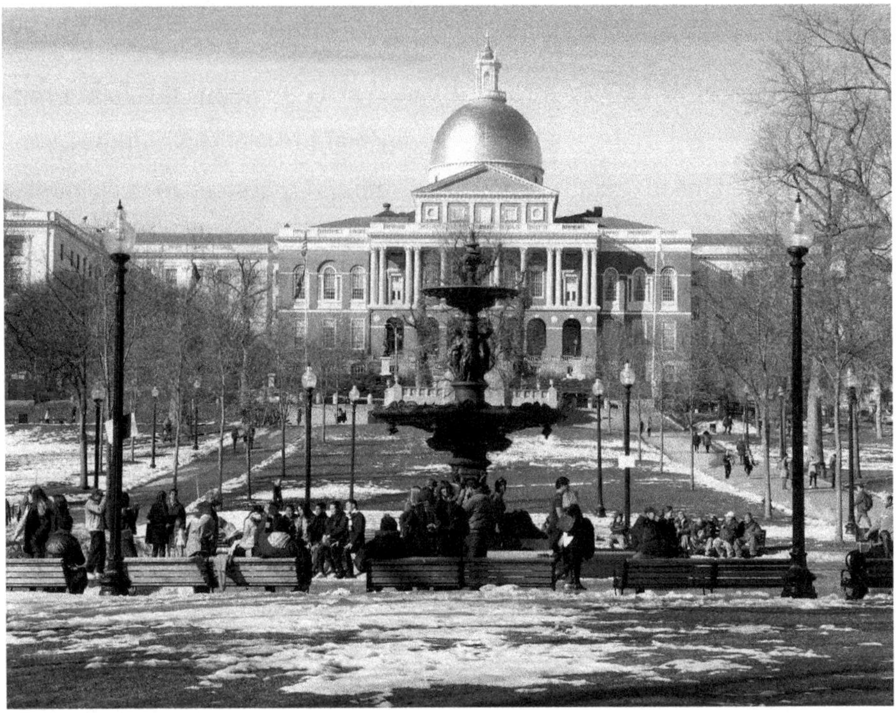

how are you today?" Today, to my complete surprise, the glass front doors swing open as we approach them. Joe walks through using his walker, and I follow. We walk toward the concierge desk and Joe beams his very best smile and thanks the concierge for opening the door and wishes him a great day. What a breakthrough this is for us, because Joe simply won't stand for anything less.

We're getting into a bit of a routine in Boston. Joe has radiation daily Monday through Friday, physical therapy twice a week, and an infusion every two weeks. And starting our second week in Boston, he has occupational therapy twice weekly to address things like his mental capacity and memory.

Judging by her face, I estimate that the occupational therapist is in her mid 30s. She's very attractive, with brown eyes and dark blond hair.

She introduces herself to us, and Joe beams his very best smile to her. She spends the next 45 minutes evaluating him, asking a series of questions and having him try a few simple memory tasks. She records his answers and says she'll review his test results with us at the next visit. When Joe excuses himself to go to the restroom, I ask her what she thinks, hoping to get some information while he's gone. She's a bit evasive until she sees how worried I am, so she decides to tell me a couple of things. First, she suspects Joe has an issue with his short-term memory, not unlike a person with early stages of dementia. Second, she doesn't know whether it'll improve over time. Part of the reason she'll be seeing Joe so frequently is so she can determine whether Joe is making progress. With brain surgery and ongoing cancer treatment, it's difficult to assess whether test results indicate a permanent condition or a temporary one. Radiation treatment in particular can lead to brain swelling that causes issues that may later subside. Her conclusions are consistent with what I've observed, but I'm encouraged that it may get better. Joe returns and we ride-share home. We're getting pretty good at this ride-sharing thing.

Joe's radiation appointments changed to 7 a.m. after the first week. I groan to myself when I find out, because he's definitely not a morning person—I know how hard it'll be to have him ready to get to the hospital so early. We adjust our schedules so that Joe takes a shower each night before he goes to bed and I have his clothes laid out and ready for him; then we'll have breakfast at the hospital after the appointment. I'm worried that I won't be able to find a ride-share driver at 6:30 a.m. to take us to the hospital, but fortunately, we get a quick response indicating that a driver will arrive in three minutes. We rush out the tall glass doors and wait on the edge of the sidewalk.

Soon an SUV approaches us and a driver that we used last week steps out. He helps Joe with his walker, and we're off to the hospital. I thank him for driving us, and I tell him I was worried we wouldn't find a driver so early in the morning. He explains that he lives nearby and that he starts working at around the same time every day. I ask him if he'd be willing to take us to MGH at the same time every day since Joe's schedule is fixed for the next five weeks. I don't really expect that he'll be able to do it, but to my surprise, he agrees. We decide on a rate, and we now have a way to get to the early appointments every day. He doesn't want us to pay him until the end of the five weeks. I can't believe our good luck, but I'm eager to see if it actually works out. The driver introduces himself as Bismarck, and Joe and I introduce ourselves.

◆

Before we left Connecticut, I'd made arrangements for Andrew, a friend of the family, to stop by our house a couple of days a week. He would feed our cats, give them fresh water, keep their litter box clean, and spend some time with them. I'd also left him some prepaid shipping envelopes so he could send our mail to us weekly.

Andrew and his parents have been friends of ours since we moved to Connecticut from Florida sixteen years ago. They lived in the same neighborhood as we did for many years, and Andrew is the same age as Greg. Joe played golf with Jim and Andrew for many years, and we'd frequently have dinner together. Cheryl and I would go for neighborhood walks, comparing our insights of Connecticut versus Florida. I was sure I could count on Andrew, as he's very dependable and responsible. And he was. He sent us our forwarded mail every Friday. I was expecting mostly bills, but to my surprise there were also many cards for Joe. Joe looks forward to getting the mail and opening his cards each week. Also, our Boston address was spread around before we knew it. There's always a card or a gift for Joe when I check our Boston mailbox every day.

Our first mail package from Andrew arrives on Tuesday, February 23. Among the bills are several get-well cards for Joe that his closest work colleagues sent. I pass them to Joe to open and read. Joe has a condition called "essential tremor,"* a disorder of the nervous system that affects his left hand from time to time. It's not associated with his glioma—he's had it all his life. Today the condition is making it challenging for him to manage the cards, so I open them and hand them to him.

The first two cards are from a couple of his work colleagues wishing him a speedy recovery. The third card is from a friend of his, Bennett, whom he hasn't heard from since his diagnosis. Bennett travels quite a bit, so it isn't uncommon for a couple of months to pass without Joe hearing from him. Greg is friends with his daughter Caitlin, so I assumed he would've heard about Joe's illness through her. Bennett included a handwritten note in the card that reads:

"Joe, wanted to check in! Hearing from Greg via Caitlin that things are going well. I understand you're headed off to Boston for a month of treatment. I know it'll be a challenge, but if it helps, we'll be thinking about you. Make sure you give us some contact info so we can stay in touch."

It also includes some information about a friend from college, plus some football talk. Bennett also talks about the series *House of Cards* and recommends it. He closes by saying:

"Let me know if you want to visit or talk on the phone. Only if it's good for you. Otherwise, I'll just drop you a note now and then. Joe, the gang loves you and is thinking about you. Let us know if we can help. Hang tough, big guy! And best to Lynn as she fights this with you! Bennett"

The card means a lot to Joe, and he reads it a couple of times. Joe and Bennett have known each other since they met as freshmen at the University of Tennessee in 1975. They lived in the same dormitory and were both engineering majors. They shared many classes, friends, sports events, and college escapades during their undergraduate days. A story about job interviewing is a favorite they both told over the years. And it's consistently been retold without too many embellishments by either one.

> Joe retrieves the mail from the mailbox in his dorm, hoping to find the paycheck from his job in the school cafeteria, and he isn't disappointed. There's one other envelope that he glances at, but he doesn't bother to open it. As he walks to his dorm room, he opens his paycheck and smiles. He plans to deposit most of the paycheck and use the remainder for going out over the next couple of weeks. Joe goes to his room and drops his mail on his desk. Glancing at the textbooks on his desk, he thinks about the homework he needs to finish before he goes to a UT basketball game later with his roommate Brian, his hometown friend Kelleghan, and Bennet. He's relieved to hear a knock on the door, happy for a diversion from the work he knows awaits.
>
> When Joe starts to open the door, Bennett pushes it wide open and enters the room exuberantly, a folded paper held high in his right hand.
>
> "Kelleghan came through with the math problem we worked on together!" he proclaims before adding teasingly. "But he made me promise not to share it with you."

He waves the paper around Joe's face, and Joe tries to snag it, unsuccessfully. "Ha-ha," Bennett taunts. Then he hands Joe the solution to the math problem and says, "Don't you tell Kelleghan I gave you this or neither of us will ever get any help again."

Joe sits at his desk and studies the problem solution, understanding the obvious answer when he sees how it's developed, nodding in understanding. Now that that's out of the way, the rest of the afternoon will be wide open.

Bennett spots the unopened envelope on Joe's desk and asks, "Hey, what does your letter say?"

"What letter?" Joe says.

Bennett picks it up and lightly taps Joe on the head with it. "This one," he replies.

Joe grabs it and asks, "What's so special about it?"

"Open it and see," quips Bennett.

Joe shrugs and tears open the envelope. As he reads, his eyes open wider. "Wow, I didn't expect this! This is great—an offer and a trip to Florida!" Joe exclaims.

"What, you have an offer? I have a trip, but no offer," Bennett says. "Let me see that." He pulls the letter from Joe's hand.

"Well, you son of a gun, you really do have an offer! I know your GPA is higher than mine, but an offer already?" Bennett says enviously. "You lucky dog—you always have it so easy."

Both of their letters request a phone call to schedule a trip to Florida to see the facility and the area. Joe and Bennett coordinate their schedules and pick a Friday to visit, intending to stay the weekend. Once the arrangements have been made, they return to their plan of finishing their homework and going to the basketball game.

A couple of weeks later, on Thursday afternoon March 13, Joe and Bennett take a flight from McGhee Tyson Airport to Palm Beach International Airport in anticipation of their all-day tours of the plant the next day. They rent cars and then drive to the Holiday Inn in Palm Beach Gardens. In the late afternoon, they visit Singer Island and sit on the beach, watching an impromptu game of coed beach volleyball. The girls were suntanned, scantily clad, enthusiastic players—quite an eyeful. Later, they have dinner at the Greenhouse restaurant and bar. They're on expense accounts for the weekend, and they're determined to make the most of it.

The next day, each has breakfast with his tour guide before taking the drive to the facility for their individual interviews with several departments. Joe is reasonably relaxed, since he already has a job offer and is very interested in the job he's considering accepting. When his tour and interviews are over, he asks his tour guide to tell Bennett to meet him in the bar for happy hour when he's finished. The tour guide gives Bennet the message, but within earshot of the employee who's wrapping up an interview with him. Bennett cringes, worried about the impression it gives the interviewer.

Later, the two meet up at an outside beachfront bar and rehash their day of interviewing. Bennett mentions many times that he's worried that he won't get an offer because of the message Joe left for him.

No worries, though, as he gets a job offer early the next week.

Bennett jokingly reminds Joe about the message and the subsequent embarrassment many times over the upcoming years.

They each eventually accept job offers at the same company and continue their friendship for many, many years.

◆

Joe's appointments for radiation, infusion immunotherapy, physical and occupational therapy, and various doctors continue as scheduled for the next five weeks. We're at MGH Monday through Friday, typically for two appointments a day. Sometimes we accomplish what we need to do in one trip, but we usually go back and forth twice. Between appointments, we fit in a walk either in the Boston Commons park or around the hospital. We know our way around the hospital pretty well now, and we start going to the hospital hair salon for Joe's haircuts. His hair has grown back enough to cover his incision, and he hasn't lost hair from the radiation. His hair was mostly gray, but it's growing back his original dark color. He often jokes that brain surgery is a cure for graying hair. Joe has always been meticulous in his personal grooming, and he continues to be so during treatment—he wants to look as normal as possible. I suppose this helps as he focuses on returning to life before surgery.

We continue with the exercises from his physical therapist, and Joe does them twice a day when he can. If there are no afternoon appointments, we walk to the Boston Commons park. This year, the average temperatures are higher and average snowfall lower than typical winters in Boston, which makes our opportunities for walking much greater. Joe isn't feeling fatigue from the radiation or the infusion treatments, and he's in a good frame of mind as we continue to follow directions from his doctors and therapists. By the third week in Boston, Joe has almost completely stopped using his walker when we go to the park, although I bring it as a precaution. We have an established routine and feel more comfortable with the logistics, and most importantly, Joe is doing well with the treatment. He's had no side effects, and he's eating well and getting stronger. We both know the path we're on is risky, but we're happy to be together.

Joe continues working with the occupational therapist, who assigns him homework to complete between visits. The homework activities include memory exercises, puzzles, reading and then reciting what he read, simple math problems, and scheduling appointments on a calendar. Joe doesn't like doing the activities, so I have to I badger him to do them. I can't tell if he thinks they're beneath him or they're hard for him to do. I ask him, but don't get a direct response.

After dinner each evening, we reach out to each other and share how we feel about so many things. We've exhausted talking about the medical care, so instead we reminisce about our time together over the years. We rehash our beliefs, whether they're religious, political, direction in our lives, and what we plan to do with our remaining time together. We dream together of leaving the northeast and moving to Florida. We'll play golf, ride bikes, walk on the beach, enjoy great food, and never wear a winter coat, gloves, or hat again. Our discussions of the future, in spite of Joe's diagnosis, help us remain positive and believe we have several years ahead of us together. We focus on what will be in our future together, and it helps us deal with the present.

On our third weekend in Boston, Joe suggests we go out for dinner, which we haven't done since Joe's surgery. It was our habit to go out for dinner once a week or so, usually on Thursday night. We worked for the same company, which had a large campus—several acres in size. Many of the campus buildings are interconnected, and you can walk for miles in the winter through the various buildings. We worked in two adjacent buildings that housed the engineering team and were connected by a second-floor walkway bridge. One of us would call the other, and we'd meet at one of our offices on our way to the parking lot. We'd follow each other to one of our favorite restaurants on the drive home. Going out for dinner was one way we stayed connected while both of us were working so much.

We don't know the Boston area, so we use our phones to look for a restaurant within walking distance from our apartment. We make reservations for 6 p.m. at No. 9 Park Street, which is within walking distance and is on our route to the Boston Commons park. It's quite cold and windy in Boston tonight, so we're bundled up for our walk to the restaurant. We arrive early, and we notice that there are very few other guests as we're seated in a small, cozy booth for two. We enjoy reading the menu—so many great choices for us. We both order without restraint and enjoy our first dinner out together since we got the news that changed our lives.

But it's a bittersweet dinner for me. As I look at Joe sitting across the table from me, I wonder how many more opportunities like this we'll have. It's amazing to me that he wanted to go out, but I believe that, like me, he's reaching for some stability in our activities by enjoying something as simple as a night out—something we used to do frequently. As optimistic as we both are, we're both seeking a path back to the life we had before Joe's diagnosis.

Over the next several weeks, Joe wants to go out a few more times. We have delicious meals at Mooo Restaurant and Grotto, both within walking distance from our rented condominium. Joe continues to become physically stronger, walking more and more each day. There are several sunny days when the temperature is in the high 50s, which bolsters our spirits and makes us feel so fortunate to have this time together.

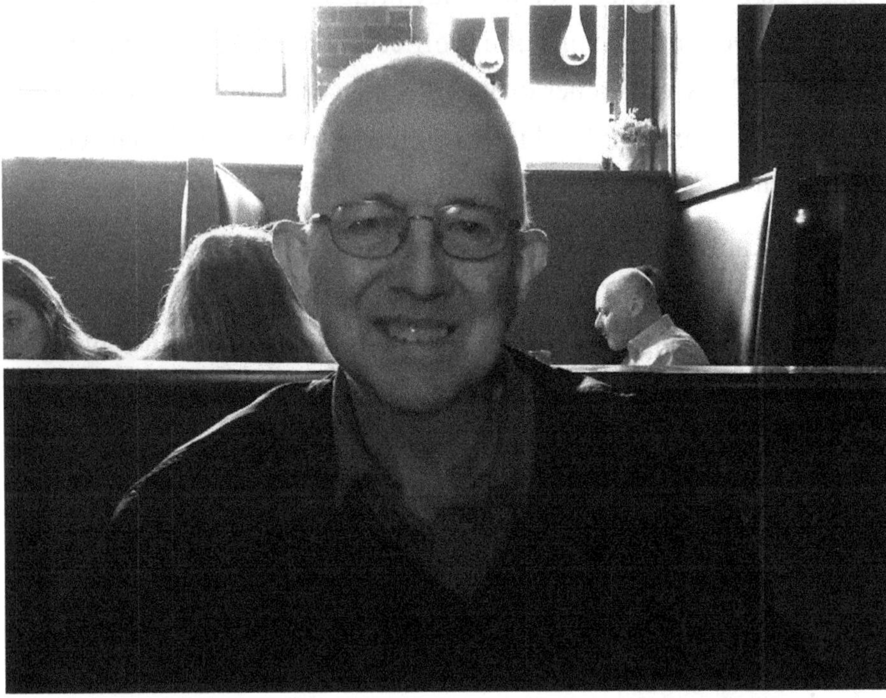

◆

During our six-week stay in Boston, Joe receives many cards from family, friends, and colleagues. He also gets several packages from his colleague Jean, including baked goods, mostly chocolate of some type. A couple of times, she sends brownies, which Joe loves. My mother and my sister Kathy also send him gifts with chocolate, knowing how much he loves it. My sister Peggy sends an extra-soft plush throw blanket with cat paws printed on it, intending that it remind Joe of his pets without making him miss them too much.

Of particular conversation was a gift my sister Kathy sent.

About halfway through our stay, a package arrives for Joe. He opens the box and out springs a large, brilliant-yellow pillow that looks like a giant Easter marshmallow chick. It's about three feet high, and it's a bit awkward to hold on to. We immediately call it "the peep pillow," and we joke about where to put it in the apartment. It's quite an eyesore, and it captures attention anywhere it's placed.

The next time Greg visits us, he immediately points at it and asks, "What is that?" We explain what it is as he throws it into the air, catches it, and then pretends to throw Joe a bullet pass. "'This is one ugly pillow!" he exclaims. When we have dinner that night, we're sure to put it on a chair, joining us at the table.

A few days later, Greg tells us his friend Bobby and his roommate Chris would like to visit Joe. Bobby and his family were our neighbors when we first moved to Connecticut. Despite being three years younger than Greg, Bobby was involved in neighborhood activities with Greg. Our houses were at the end of a cul-de-sac, ours on the right and Bobby's centered. Across the street was a family with four children, including one boy who's older than Greg and another who's Greg's age. The four boys found lots of things do together over the summer and during the school year, like bike riding, in-line skating, lacrosse, street hockey, and sledding. We had a finished basement with a pool table that could be converted to table tennis, which the boys often used during the winter. Of course, there were also video games at everyone's house.

From the time Bobby was young, he was very definitive in his opinion about many subjects, and he was never afraid to express those opinions. The neighborhood houses were typically on one-acre lots. During the summer, families spent time caring for their lawns, most using lawn tractors. We had a 22-hp lawn tractor, and Joe was known as the neighborhood tractor racer. He would get on the lawn tractor and drive up and down the lawn, cutting the grass in straight lines as much as he could until he approached a tree. Then he would circle the tree, sometimes going so fast you would think tractor would flip over. It never did, but parents and children alike would stare as he cut around trees. When Bobby would visit, he would comment on Joe's tractor driving, making it clear he felt it was unnecessary to drive that way.

Both Bobby and Greg ended up with jobs in Boston when they graduated from college. They reconnected after graduation, and they're still friends today. When Bobby found out about Joe's diagnosis, he knew how serious it was because he works for a hospital insurance company. He wanted to visit Joe to wish him well and spend some time with him.

Chris and Greg are roommates in Boston, and they were friends in high school. Chris has been to our house many times over the years, and Joe always has conversations with Chris when he visits, usually about inane life topics. Joe, Greg, Chris, and Bobby have played many table tennis games over the years, with plenty of trash talk throughout the game. Chris has also been very kind in letting us stay at their apartment while we sorted out Joe's treatment options.

Bobby and Greg arrive at the condo at around 5:30 p.m. after finishing work for the day.

"Hey, Mr. G! How are you doing?" Bobby says. "Good to see you!"

Joe stands and shakes Bobby's hand.

"I'm not sure I would've recognized you if I saw you walking by," Joe says to him. "You're dressed so well and have a different haircut! Quite the man about town!" Joe comments.

"I'm doing well and so glad to see you," Bobby replies.

Bobby takes a seat and immediately notices the peep pillow in the chair across from him.

"What's that?" he asks, pointing, and we tell him the amusing story.

There's a knock on the door, and Greg opens it and welcomes Chris in.

"Mr. Gambill, how are you doing?" Chris says.

"So glad to see you, Chris, and thanks for letting us stay at the apartment—it was a big help to us," Joe replies.

Chris sits on the opposite end of the couch from Joe, and Greg pulls up a dinette chair. The tiny living room is crowded. I go to the kitchen and stand in the pass-through to be part of the gathering. Chris notices the peep pillow, and before you know it, he, Greg, and Bobby are playing catch with it. They continue their game while Bobby explains how he found a job in Boston and Chris talks about his job. They talk about the upcoming presidential election and have many differing opinions on the subject. They also compare the Boston area to Connecticut, agreeing that it's so much better to be in Boston. So much more to do, an exciting big city with so many people to meet.

The topic of dating comes up, and Bobby and Chris talk about their current girlfriends and how they met. Joe starts giving them dating advice in a joking way, saying things like "Do they pay their share when you go out on dates? Well, they really should!" and "I hope you choose where you want to go. Be sure they know you're in charge!" Lots of eye rolling and smiles from all three boys as Joe offers his dating wisdom. I'm more of an observer than a participant in this visit, except to be sure the guests have something to drink.

I can't help but feel overwhelmed and touched that Bobby and Chris want to spend time with Joe. These young men are 26 and 27 years old, and there are so many other things they could be doing tonight.

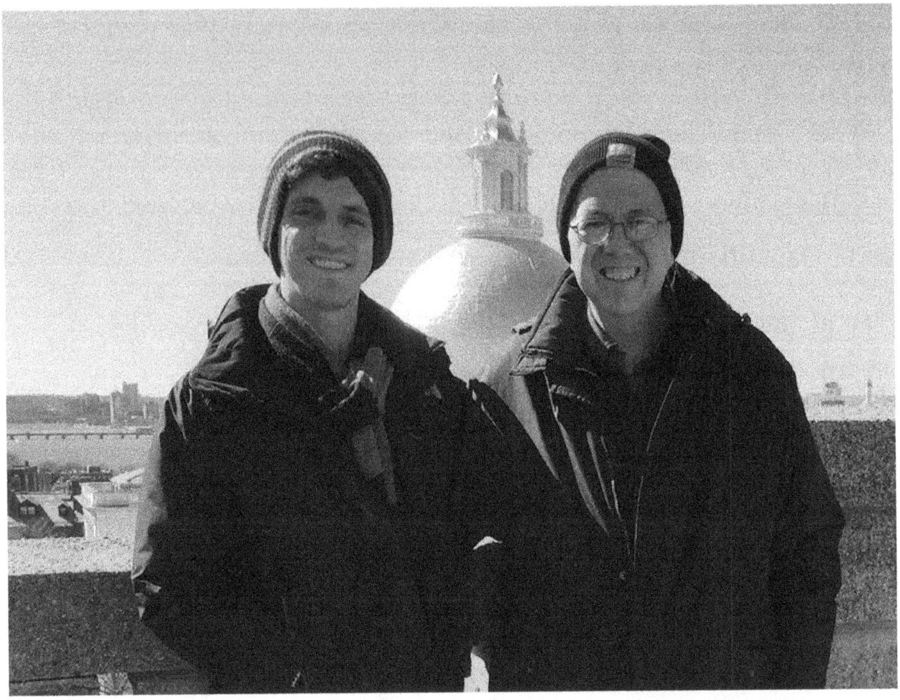

But they want to be with Joe, talk and joke with him. They comment on the condo and Joe stands to lead a tour. He shows them the airplane-size bathroom and the tiny bedroom. The tour takes all of three minutes. Then Joe reminds us that the Airbnb ad says there's a rooftop sitting area with outdoor seating that overlooks the State Capitol dome. So we decide to explore as a group.

We walk downstairs to the 10th floor and across a short corridor to a door labeled "outside grill." We use our key to open the door and enter a rooftop area furnished with white patio chairs, brown wood benches, and matching tables. There's an outdoor grill as claimed in the ad, but there's also an indoor kitchen area. The patio overlooks the State Capitol dome and has a beautiful view of the Boston Commons park and the surrounding area. Winter is still in full force, with a blustery wind and 40-degree temperature. We're bundled up and decide to take a few pictures, but we don't stay outside very long.

Bobby, Chris, and Greg are planning to stop in at a couple of local establishments after they leave, so they say their goodbyes. Joe is the perfect host, walking them to the elevator and wishing them a good time.

When Joe returns, he sits on the couch and says, "You know, Lynn, that was such a nice time, and I'm so surprised that they wanted to see us. They're all grown up and are doing so well. I'm so proud of all of them." Then he's quiet, and I sit with him on the couch, equally impressed.

The fifth week we're in Boston, Greg meets us for dinner at a restaurant called 75 Chestnut Street, about three-quarters of a mile away. Joe is able to walk from our condo all the way to the restaurant, resting only once along the way, and it takes us about 20 minutes. Greg joins Joe and me soon after we're seated. It's a major event for the three of us to celebrate Joe's progress together.

Next week, Joe's radiation therapy comes to an end, and we're so happy it's almost over. Joe continues to have very few side effects and is happier and stronger every day. We have dinner together and discuss Boston, Greg's job, what he's been doing, and our plans to return to Connecticut. We're thankful for the many things people have done to help us during our stay. We walk together through the park back to our home in Boston, Joe and Greg walking several feet ahead. The two of them are so comfortable talking with each other, and Joe occasionally jabs Greg's shoulder playfully in response to whatever comment Greg makes.

Joe completed 30 radiation sessions and three infusion treatments while we were in Boston. In addition, there were many physical and occupational therapy appointments and doctor visits. On the day of his last radiation treatment, our driver Bismarck takes us to MGH again. He's been driving us to the hospital for four weeks, and we've become fond of him. We thank him for taking such good care of us each morning, and we wish him well. Bismarck knows about Joe's diagnosis and tells us that he'll continue to pray for him. He hands us his business card, and we learn that he's actually a clergyman but works for the ride-share service for extra income. That explains a lot.

As Joe completes his last radiation treatment, he thanks the team who worked with him. They learned what music he likes, and they always played his favorites during his treatment. They give him his radiation mask to take with him, shake his hand, and wish him the best before they walk him to a bell affixed to the wall near the radiation waiting area. They all watch as Joe rings the bell, as is customary for patients to do to signify that they're moving to the next step in recovery. Those in the waiting room applaud, as it's a major move forward in treatment.

On the morning of March 30, 2016, we leave Boston and return to Connecticut. The car is packed with fewer things than we brought with us, keeping every card and gift Joe received except for the peep pillow, which Greg and his friends "adopted." It's a clear, sunny day in the 50s as we drive home. We're excited to be returning home and feel that so much has been accomplished. Joe is walking unassisted, hasn't felt the effects of radiation, has no side effects from the infusion treatments, and is in good spirits. There are so many people who helped us during this time, and we're so grateful for people's generosity. As we leave the building, the concierge smiles and waves at us, wishing us well.

Chapter 5: Planning Ahead

Wild men who caught and sang the sun in flight,
And learn, too late, they grieved it on its way,
Do not go gentle into that good night.

Dylan Thomas

We managed to adapt to our rental in Boston and the treatment regimen while trying to establish a sense of normalcy in an abnormal state of affairs. We're anxious to be back in our home in Connecticut, in a familiar environment with our possessions in their proper places. When I drive the car into the garage, I'm quick to park. So fast, in fact, that Joe quips, "Watch it, Weather!" in reference to a character in John Sanford's novels about Detective Lucas Davenport. In one of the books, Davenport's wife Weather accidentally rams her Porsche into the garage door because she's too fast driving. It made a lasting impression on Joe, and he's lambasted me with the comment many times that I've driven into our garage. I scowl, snicker a little, and say, "There was nothing to worry about!" But I do appreciate that he remembers to say it.

Joe is capable of getting out of the car, walking up the two short steps to the garage side door end entering our house unassisted. He walks into the sunroom and takes a seat. Almost instantaneously, he's accosted by our two cats, Rascal and Simba, as they meow and purr loudly. They jump on the sofa, surround Joe, and tussle for the best position to sit in his lap. They each find a satisfying location, and Joe pets and comforts them, talking to them in a soft voice. As he keeps the cats occupied, I unpack the car and reinstate our travel items to their proper places.

Andrew had done a great job of taking care of the cats and the house, and I so appreciate his help. Rascal and Simba are well fed and happy, and their litter box is clean. It looks like the sunroom has been vacuumed to keep cat litter from spreading around the house, which I assume Andrew did. I open the silhouette window shades so light will shine into the room. It's a beautiful sunny afternoon, so the room gets warm quickly. Joe and the cats are snoozing soon after.

I review the food situation in the pantry and refrigerator and make a list of what we need. There's a grocery store a five-minute drive from our house, so I nudge Joe to let him know my plans before I leave. Because I worked and managed our household for years, I acquired what I term "drive-by shopping" skills. With a shopping list handy and being familiar with the store layout, I can zip through the store and get everything I need in about fifteen minutes. I have further refined this skill since Joe first got ill. I don't want to be away from him for any length of time in case he needs me, so I'm back to the house 30 minutes after I leave.

I walk to the kitchen and unload the groceries without disturbing Joe and the cats. Then I take a seat in the TV room, which overlooks the sunroom. My mind is so busy, spinning with the many tasks that need to be done. I start formulating methods for doing each task, knowing I'll have to write things down so I don't miss anything. For now, I'll let things percolate in my mind. Soon, I too, nod off.

While I sleep, I dream about Joe. In my mind, he looks like he's in his mid 40s and is wearing golf clothes. He walks to the garage door in the house we lived in before we moved to Connecticut. He turns to me and smiles and waves, and I wish him a good game. He opens the garage door and steps down into the garage. But the garage floor is underwater, with the water swirling around. Joe tries to walk through the water to get in his car as if nothing is unusual. I walk to the doorway and peer out as Joe opens the outside garage door. It looks as if the garage door was holding back a wall of water 10 feet high, and with the door now open, the water forcefully rushes into the garage. Joe is soon up to his waist in water, and I'm watching him from the doorway. I call out to Joe and try to step into the garage, but something is preventing me from going in. I keep pushing and pushing, desperately trying to get in, but I can't move past the doorway. I watch the water continue to rise, now as high as Joe's shoulders. He starts moving around the garage, the water lifting him into the swirl. Round and round he goes, his head up as he tries to breathe. The water starts rushing out of the garage, with Joe trapped as if he's in an undertow. I watch helplessly as he's swept out of the garage, his head up and arms flailing. I wake up, startled and feeling very unsettled. The final image of Joe in the water sticks in my mind. I know it was only a dream, but I feel so uneasy. I get up, go into the sunroom, and see that Joe is still sleeping on the sofa. I sit on the floor next to him. I reach out and place my hand on his arm, and I hold on while he sleeps.

◆

Now that we're home in Connecticut, we start a new routine. Joe wakes up at around 8:30 a.m., showers (with me close by), and eats a prepared breakfast. He takes his e-reader into the sunroom and reads the local newspaper. He also texts his friends and colleagues. At around 11 a.m. or sometime after lunch, I usually drive us to Nevers Park in South Windsor. With more than two miles of walking trails, there are several routes we can choose from depending on how far Joe wants to walk. Each route has different things to see, such as a dog park, a soccer field, baseball fields, and cornfields. Every time we go, we decide whether to start with an incline or a decline, depending on how Joe feels. We're both eager to continue the walking routine we developed in Boston, because it was very rewarding and helped improve Joe's strength and capability. He enjoys being outside and loves it when there are dogs at the park. He likes to sit on the bench outside the park and watch the dogs play.

Without his physical therapist from MGH to guide him, Joe isn't very motivated to complete the exercises she instructed him to continue with. I try every day to persuade him to do them, and some days he does, while other days he refuses. He enjoys walking, but he isn't pushing himself to walk farther.

I don't particularly like this turn of events, so I call Dr. W, his primary care physician. Dr. W suggests we continue with physical and occupational therapy until Joe has fully recovered. I like that idea, because Joe seems to respond when a therapist works with him. The doctor recommends a facility that's about 40 minutes away, but he says it's "the best in the state" for physical and occupational therapy. It takes a couple of weeks for our insurance carrier to approve the request and for the facility to contact us for Joe's first therapy sessions. Like choosing MGH for Joe's treatment, we continue to try to get the best treatment for him. If it means driving farther, we'll do it.

In the meantime, we continue with our walking routine, and Joe sometimes does his exercises at home, albeit reluctantly. I constantly remind him that the exercises are important for his strength so he can return to work. We occasionally walk around our small neighborhood, and we sometimes see our neighbors along the way. We've lived in this home for seven years, and we're friendly with several of the neighbors. They became aware of Joe's condition when Joe returned after his surgery and recovered for a month at home before we moved to Boston. The couples we see most frequently on our walks are Ray and Lynette, Ray and Kathy, and Ben and Glenna. They've all stopped by our home to see how Joe is doing and to offer any help they can.

After our daily walks, we have lunch and Joe rests for a couple of hours. While Joe relaxes, I prepare for the things Joe and I agreed to do. The list is long and includes finishing our 2015 tax return, wills, Joe's advance care directive, his "do not resuscitate" document, his closure with his siblings on his parents' estate, financial advisor meetings, selling our house in Connecticut, selling our second house in Florida, retirement decision, many insurance issues, Joe's work status, and coordinating his siblings' visits. All these things are to be completed around Joe's infusion treatment schedule and therapy sessions. It's a daunting task list, and I'm exhausted just writing everything down.

I use a combined calendar planner notebook to start figuring out a schedule for all the things we want to do. The first things I write in it are Joe's treatment requirements. Then I schedule appointments with our CPA, our attorney, and our financial advisor. Typically, we file our own tax return, with Joe compiling the information and filling out the forms. Obviously, we need a different approach, so we hired a CPA to help us this year. While Joe was recovering from his surgery and before we went to Boston for radiation treatment, I collected the necessary information and delivered it to a CPA. The next step is for us to meet with the CPA, review the form, and sign it. Our wills are partially complete, but we need to meet with our attorney to update, sign, and file them. Our financial advisor will meet with us to discuss our status and determine whether my early retirement would be financially feasible. Joe needs someone to be with him during the day, and we have to weigh this cost versus my retiring to be with him. I don't want to hire someone—I prefer to be with him every minute that I can. I still really don't know how much time he has, and I don't want to miss any opportunity to spend it with him. Unknown to Joe, I've already decided to do this regardless of the financial advice, but I'd like to understand what the implications will be.

The first two weeks we're home from Boston, we're very busy with Joe's walking, exercising, resting, and various appointments. We go to our CPA's office and have our taxes filed, we meet with our attorney, and we meet with our financial advisor in our home. Joe drafts a letter to his brother and sister to finish his duties as his parents' estate executor, which I type up on the computer for him. These activities are tiring for Joe, and they're spread out over a couple of weeks. We're both unhappy with ourselves for not already having finalized things like our wills, Joe's parents' estate, and a more detailed financial evaluation earlier in our lives. We really don't have an excuse other than that we thought we'd have more time. Lesson to us: you never know when your life will be turned upside-down. Our taxes couldn't have been done earlier—it was just unfortunate timing. We were also caught in the middle of buying and selling homes in Florida when Joe was diagnosed. We signed with a real estate agent to sell our Florida home in December and listed it in early January. We couldn't have avoided that, either, but it certainly adds stress to an already very difficult time in our lives.

Joe has infusion treatment every two weeks and an MRI every two months, so Greg asks us to stay with him in his apartment when we're in Boston for treatment so the three of us can spend more time together. Joe and I are so touched, and we agree. In the middle of April, we drive to Boston for Joe's MRI and infusion, which is a two-day process. The MRI, which is scheduled for 9 a.m. of the first day, is the first one since his brain surgery and radiation treatment, so we're eager yet apprehensive about the test results.

◆

On April 13, we drive to Boston earlier than usual, leaving the house at around 6 a.m. The drive into Boston isn't too bad, as we're early enough not to be snaggled in the Boston work traffic. The MRI equipment at MGH is overbooked, so we'll be shuttled to a facility in Chelsea that's affiliated with the hospital. I'm apprehensive about the change, so I tried unsuccessfully to have the MRI taken at MGH. We're familiar with the logistics at MGH—what to expect, what to plan for, and how to time it so Joe can rest at Greg's apartment if he needs to. The process for going to Chelsea seems much more exhausting, but we have no choice.

Our plan is to drive to Greg's apartment after the MRI, arriving early afternoon to give Joe time to rest before his daily walk—this time in Brookline. Spring hasn't arrived yet, so the trees are barren and the grass is brown but there's no snow on the ground. Along the way, Joe and I talk about work as we continue to be in touch with day-to-day requirements. Joe occasionally receives text messages and e-mails consulting him, I'm in contact regularly as well. We both miss the industry we've worked in for close to 40 years each, and we're staying as close as we can.

We're meeting a shuttle van at MGH at 8:15 a.m. to take us to Chelsea for Joe's MRI. After I park the car, I have some difficulty finding the van—I assumed it would be at the main entrance, but it's actually at the Yawkey Building instead. We're the only passengers in the van, and we enjoy the scenic drive to Chelsea as it's a clear morning with excellent visibility as we ride on Route 1 over the Mystic River.

The facility itself has a half dozen patients in the waiting area when we check in. I give Joe a half dose of the sedative, remembering what happened after the last MRI. The MRI proceeds on time and as expected. When it's finished, Joe is a little loopy, but the sedative hasn't affected him nearly as much as it did when he had the previous MRI. The van driver waited for us, so we leave for MGH as soon as Joe is released. My concerns about having the MRI performed in Chelsea prove to be unfounded, and the entire process, although it was longer due to travel time, was well organized. Finally, we get our car from the parking garage and drive to Greg's apartment in Brookline.

We arrive at Greg's apartment as planned, and Joe walks unassisted, slowly and carefully, up the Chattahoochee pebbled sidewalk to the front door of the apartment complex. We call Greg and let him know we've arrived so he can remotely unlock the main door and let us in. We take the elevator to the second floor, where we exit and arrive at Greg's apartment door on the right. Greg and his roommate Chris share a two-bedroom, two-bathroom apartment in a Brookline residential neighborhood. There's a reasonably sized common TV area with an overlooking kitchen. Chris is traveling, so Joe and I will sleep in his room. I brought sheets and towels from home for us to use, so I remove Chris's bedding and replace it with mine while Joe sits on the couch to watch TV.

When I return to the TV area, Joe is struggling to figure out the remote control. He hands it to me with a questioning look in his eyes. I'm surprised at that, as Joe has always been the one who manages "all things electrical." In fact, if I try to use the remote control, I usually get a verbal "smack down." Okay, something new here. I find the station Joe wants to watch and hand the remote back to him. But now he isn't interested, and he sets it on the couch next to him. With Joe safely situated, I return to our car to get our suitcase and the food I brought for our dinner and breakfast. Joe and I take a walk around the streets of Brookline. When Greg joins us after work, he orders a Thai dinner to be delivered. We have a relaxing time talking with him, sharing in his life for a night in Boston.

Greg has changed from his work clothes into his workout clothes. After Joe is in bed, Greg makes us a couple of smoothies—his with protein powder added, mine without—and heads out to the nearby gym. I watch TV, using the time to process the day's events. I'm reading a brochure I found in the waiting room earlier, published by the National Institute of Neurological Disorders and Strokes (NINDS). It's about brain basics and explains the brain architecture, noting that more than 50 million people in the US suffer from damage to the nervous system. It says NINDS supports research on more than 600 neurological diseases, including brain tumors. I scan for information about the frontal lobes, and the brochure explains that they're situated directly behind the forehead. According to the brochure, the frontal lobes are involved in tasks like planning a schedule, imagining the future, or reasoning. It says the lobes act as short-term storage sites, allowing a person to keep one idea in mind while considering others.* I mull that around and think about Joe's behavior since his surgery. He does seem less inclined to plan or schedule or remember simple logistics on a day-to-day basis. He does seem to be logical and follow and contribute to decision making. But on a daily task level, not so much. I think about the remote control. He's always been very skilled with things like that, but today, using Greg's equipment, he wasn't. He's used Greg's remote control before with no problem. I don't want to make too much of it, but I don't know whether it's significant. I decide to ask Dr. D when we meet with him tomorrow.

Greg returns after an hour or so and makes another meal—this time a vegetable stir-fry dinner—and eats so fast that you'd think he poured the food down his throat. When he's finished, he sits on the couch with me.

"So, Mom, how are you doing with all this?" he asks.

I'm looking straight ahead at the TV, and I think carefully before I answer. On the one hand, I want to protect Greg and not discuss too much with him, even though he's 26 years old. On the other hand, he's an intelligent, responsible person, and we need to communicate as openly as possible about what's happening in our family. We need to support each other as we try to adapt to the changes. So I tell him I'm doing okay and am trying to do whatever it takes to help Joe as much as I can—to be his health advocate and caregiver but still try to gauge when to push him and when to back off.

"I don't always get it right, but I'm finding my way," I tell him. "Sometimes I'm up and sometimes I'm almost panicked thinking about losing your dad. I struggle with not knowing what will happen, and I feel so unprepared, you know what I mean? Everything is on the fly, and I'm trying to figure out what to do next."

I tell him I'm anxious about the results of today's MRI and will tell him what we find out as soon as we know.

"Your dad is himself most of the time, but then the day-to-day forgetfulness will be there," I continue. "Have you noticed?"

Greg is watching me closely. "Not as much as I think you do, because you're with him all the time. But yeah, I do notice it with little things," he replies. "But you know, Dad has always been a little relaxed with timing and schedules and things like that. When he gets tired, I notice it more. He's not as strong as he used to be."

I look down at the couch we're sitting on. It's a sectional pit couch in a chambray blue fabric. We both have our feet propped up on the matching ottoman. Joe and I bought this couch for Greg when he graduated from law school. I remember shopping for it, finding it, and then bringing Joe to the store to look at it with me. At first he didn't like it. After he tried it out, he decided it was comfortable enough and a decent bargain, so we bought it. It's now two years old. My eyes tear up remembering the shopping experience. Who would've thought that so soon after we bought the couch, we'd be visiting Greg with Joe so very sick? I reach out and place my hand over Greg's, just for a moment. It's so reassuring to me that he's here.

"You know your father is so proud of you and really loves being around you," I tell him. "He always looks forward to seeing you, even under these conditions. I don't know how his disease will progress, but I think you should talk to your dad as much as you can about anything that's on your mind. He has so much experience and can give you insight into any subject.

"I know you both get along so well, but it's hard to know what's in front of us," I continue. "So try to use your time with him wisely."

Greg nods his head in response, and I can see his eyes are misty.

◆

It's Wednesday, and our schedule for the day includes Joe's bloodwork at 9 a.m., discussion with Nurse N at 9:45, an appointment with Dr. D at 10:30, and an immunotherapy infusion at 11:30. With any luck, the infusion will be complete by 3 p.m. and we'll leave the Boston area before the rush hour. We leave Greg's apartment at the same time Greg leaves for work, and he helps me bring our suitcase, sheets, and towels to the car. As Joe is about to get into the car, he turns to Greg and gives him a man hug. "Go get 'em," he says, telling Greg he'll text him later about the test results. Greg wishes him luck, and we go our separate ways.

We take the usual route to the hospital, park in the parking garage, and walk to Dr. D's office on the 9th floor of the Yawkey Building. It'll be Joe's fifth infusion, and we know the routine by now. Shortly after we check in and Joe is seated, he's called to have blood drawn. We've been told that the purpose of the blood test is to assess if he's had any negative response to the infusion and see how his immune system is responding to the treatment, which could indicate whether the treatment is working. The results can also help his doctors determine whether his treatment should stop, be modified, or continue as is.* We'd be told at each visit if there were a negative response, but per the guidelines of the clinical trial, we're not told whether the treatment seems to be working.

After Joe's blood is drawn, we wait for close to 30 minutes in the patient waiting area and then are asked to move to a patient office. We wait there for a few minutes before we're joined by Nurse N, who's been Joe's attending nurse since he began the immunotherapy treatment. Thanks to Joe's efforts, we've gotten to know her. Joe notices she has a nice dress on instead of her usual scrubs and white coat. Joe compliments her appearance and asks if today is a special occasion. She smiles back and says she and her husband are meeting her college roommate after work for drinks and dinner. She explains that she hasn't seen her roommate in many years and is looking forward to seeing her.

"Oh, and is your husband as interested? Sounds like he's a good sport!" Joe jokes.

Nurse N laughs and says her husband is okay with going. Then she starts Joe's physical exam.

The exam is routine: a check of Joe's eyes, left and right hand fingertip to nose with eyes closed, arm and leg reflexes while sitting, walk on toes and heels, walk normally and arm swing checked. Nurse N reports that all these tests show normal results. Then she rolls herself to a computer in the corner, where she looks up the results of Joe's blood tests. She scans the results, comparing each value to a reference range. The blood test includes comprehensive LDH, comprehensive metabolic panel, and CBC with differential.* She tells us the blood test results are within acceptable ranges with nothing to suggest today's infusion shouldn't proceed. With this information, we're now waiting for Dr. D to arrive and review the MRI results with us. I quickly decide to discuss with Nurse N our possible plans for my retirement and moving to Florida while we continue with Joe's treatment at MGH via air travel.

"We're assessing what we should do since Joe's surgery, and we're struggling to understand the longevity of his illness," I tell her. "Can you give us any insight so we can try to decide what to do?"

I know I'm being very direct and putting her on the spot, but we really need help with this. She isn't very surprised by the question, so I assume she's been asked all kinds of things in her job.

"I've seen patients spend a couple of years together with a glioma diagnosis and have seen others have six months or less," she replies. "It's hard to know what lies ahead."

She explains that the science of the clinical trial Joe is in is being studied and may be successful, and that a couple of patients in the study reached twelve months. She notes that Joe is healthy and tolerating the treatment well, though we can't guarantee what the upcoming months will bring.

"What are you considering?" Nurse N asks.

"I'm thinking about retiring, and then we'd move to Florida and travel back to MGH for treatment twice a month," I say. "We're trying to decide on the timing."

She pauses thoughtfully before she replies, "If you can afford to retire, I would do so if I were in your position. Then you have the most quality time with Joe."

She says several patients have moved and continue to travel twice monthly for treatment, and it seems to be working out. I have a few more questions for her, but I'm interrupted when the door opens and Dr. D walks in.

Dr. D begins by apologizing for being a little late. He explains that he was in a triage meeting with Dr. O and Dr. N, reviewing the results of Joe's MRI. Pleasantries are exchanged all around, and then Dr. D starts explaining how the brain may behave after radiation. He talks about how brain swelling can make an MRI hard to interpret, but that Joe's MRI shows signs consistent with post-operative changes. It indicates that the bones and soft tissue are stable. It also shows an area of grayness in the scan that might be either a product of the radiation or a sign of progression (growth) of the tumor. It may also indicate pseudo-progression, meaning it looks like tumor progression but actually shows a positive response to the treatment. He notes that he doesn't feel it indicates tumor progression. He recommends that Joe continue with his immunotherapy treatment based on the results of the blood tests and that we revisit the treatment after the next MRI, which is scheduled for June. I don't realize that I was probably holding my breath the entire time he talked until I exhale and feel the tightness in my chest relax. If the results of the blood tests continue to be favorable, Joe's treatment can continue for another two months—what great news!

Dr. D and Nurse N tell us we can proceed to the infusion area. As they leave the room, Joe and I make eye contact and smile broadly. Yes!!!

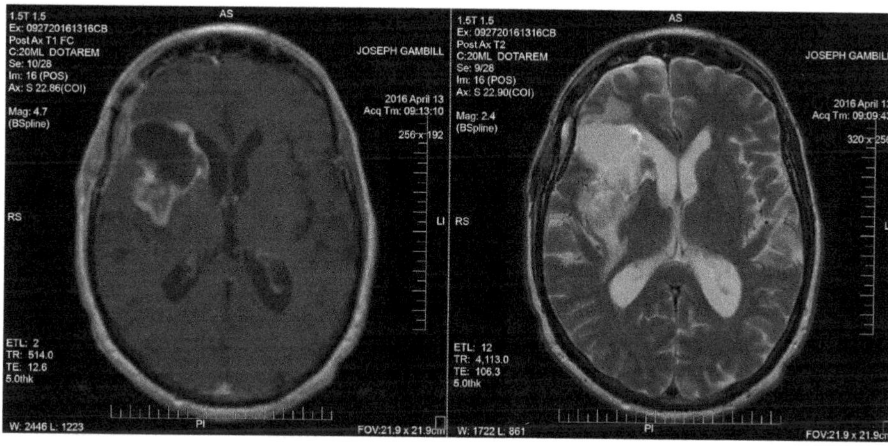

Joe and I head to the 8th floor of the Yawkey Building, going down the flight of stairs to the left of the double glass doors of the doctor's office. We check in and take seats in the waiting area, and we're ushered into the infusion area rather quickly even though we're late for the appointment. Then Joe is weighed and the information is sent to the pharmacist for the proper infusion dose to be calculated and mixed. Then we're led by an orderly to the end of a corridor where there are windows overlooking the Charles River. Joe is directed to a reclining chair from which he has a spectacular view of the many boats anchored, motoring, or sailing in the water. It's midday with the unshielded sun high overhead, which creates a twinkling reflection in the waves as they're swept by the wind. The water vessels are rocking slightly, their sails rippling as they traverse the river. Each infusion area is separated with curtains mounted to a rail attached to the ceiling. Only those next to the windows can see the river, unless the curtains are open.

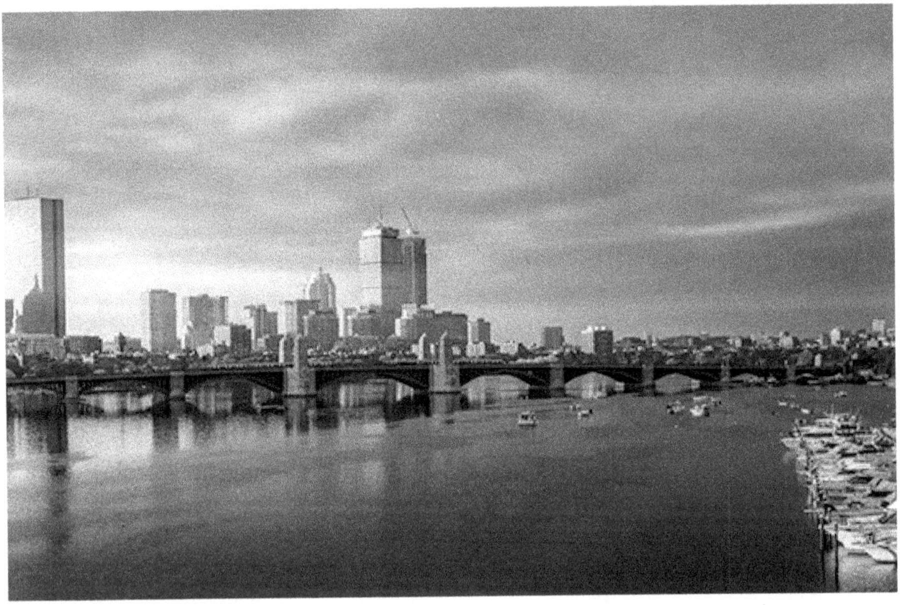

Joe has an assigned infusion nurse, who started with him on his third treatment and will be his nurse for the duration of his immunotherapy. She's always pleasant, with an easy composure and unperturbed perspective. She's close to 5'8" tall, with a medium build, long, slightly wavy dark hair, blue eyes, and a fair complexion. She has a strong Boston accent, and she smiles a lot. We know she has two daughters and works four days a week—usually ten-hour days. She's a breath of fresh air to us each time she helps Joe, always trying to make the process as easy as possible. She knows we're trying to leave the hospital no later than 3:30 p.m. so we aren't caught in the heavy traffic leaving the city, so she does what she can to help us. But the exact schedule isn't in her control, as the pharmacy schedule determines how long it takes to mix the medicine. Today, it arrives about an hour and half after Joe is seated and the infusion process takes about an hour and a half. Joe's nurse removes the IV* carefully. It's one of the only things he reacts to during his treatment, always asking that the IV be removed with care. She obliges, and Joe relaxes and tells her, "Good job!" We both thank her before we leave, eager to be on the road home.

It's a long day for Joe, so I push him in the wheelchair. We take the elevator from the 8th floor of the Yawkey Building to the 2nd floor and continue through corridors to the Lunder Building elevator. When the elevator doors open, a wheelchair pushed by a man perhaps in his early 60s exits. In the wheelchair is a man in his early 30s or so, and there's a long incision with staples holding the skin together on the left side of his head. He looks quite haggard, his skin grayish and his face unshaven. "Oh no, another patient with recent brain surgery," I think to myself. My heart goes out to this younger man as I understand what he must be going through. We aren't able to make eye contact, because they're exiting quickly, but Joe says, "Hang in there, it gets easier." The older man acknowledges with a head nod, and we exchange places in the elevator. That's the first patient we've seen with something that appears to be similar to Joe's condition.

After I get the car from the parking garage, pick Joe up at the hospital main entrance, and begin the drive home to Connecticut. We leave the hospital at 4 p.m. and struggle through the traffic leaving Boston. It takes a little more than two hours to drive home, and Joe sleeps most of the drive. I call Greg and explain the MRI results. He's also so happy to know the treatment is continuing.

I decide we should rest for the day between the trip home from Boston and Joe's first appointment with the new therapy care hospital in Connecticut. It's on our day off that we receive the good news that an offer was made on our house in Florida. The house was on the market for a little over four months, and I'd been worried about selling it. The offer was reasonable, and we accepted. We'll need to remove our furnishings, personal effects, automobile, kitchen items, pictures, and electronics from the home in time for the closing date in the middle of May. In December, I arranged for a moving company to relocate our items to the home in Florida farther north, but the items would need to be boxed up first.

Once again, my sister Peggy comes to my rescue and volunteers to pack everything up and to coordinate with the movers. Because this is our second home, there are fewer personal items than there'd be in a full-time residence, but it's a big undertaking nonetheless. Peggy buys boxes, packing paper, tape, box markers, electrical wire labels, and whatever else is needed and sends me the receipts for repayment. She has an extra-large SUV that can be used to move fragile items. She offers to manage the move, and I feel so indebted to her for her kindness, knowing that it's an extraordinary sacrifice she's making to help us out. There's more work to do than pack up the house. For example, when pictures are removed from the wall, any marks or holes need to be cleaned, spackled, and painted. Peggy offers to do all of that, in addition to thoroughly cleaning the house before the final inspection. If you've ever moved, you know what a chore that is. And to do it for someone else is amazingly generous.

I'm so humbled and thankful to have the help when we're so desperate handling Joe's illness. Not knowing what the illness was really about, I had no idea that the path we were on relocating homes would be something I'd have such difficulty trying to do myself. My plan was to have Greg stay with Joe while I flew to Florida to handle it. Peggy's help will allow me to stay with Joe and carry on the caregiver support he needs and be with him as much as I can. I cry all afternoon with relief, knowing Peggy will handle the move and overwhelmed that she's willing to do so much.

◆

Friday is Joe's first appointment with the facility Dr. W recommended for his therapy. It's an assessment appointment to determine the type and frequency of therapy he'll need, and it's scheduled for 4 p.m. I take I-84W passing through downtown Hartford, just missing the weekend exodus. Joe often says the area is "not a destination city," meaning people leave the area to go on vacation, hence the weekend exodus. It's a 45-minute drive from the door to the parking lot, and we have high expectations as I park the car. The facility is a reasonable size, newer looking than most buildings in the area. It appears to have attached lodging, presumably hospital rooms. We go through glass sliding doors and turn right past a grand piano into a patient seating area. There are five glass-enclosed patient check-in stations, one of which is occupied by a staff member who checks Joe in. He's the only patient in the waiting area, I assume because it's late on a Friday afternoon.

We wait 20 minutes or so before we're asked to follow an employee who walks us to a double-door entryway, which she activates with a badge hanging around her neck, then leads us through a patient therapy room. We take seats at a rectangular laminate table opposite a therapist I'll refer to as "S." Behind S are open shelves with several baskets filled with what look like physical therapy aids. She starts Joe's evaluation by asking about his medical history and current medications. She then assesses his physical capability through a series of hand-eye coordination tests, strength tests, and walking tests. She also tests his cognitive level. He answers questions and fills out simple exercise sheets she gives him. Then she tests his short-term memory by telling him a name, an address, and a type of animal; talking to him about various other things for five minutes; and then asking him to repeat the three items. He can remember the name only. She asks him the time and day, and she notes that he uses his watch to answer. She shows him a few mathematical figures and asks him to connect lines to match shapes and do simple arithmetic, like adding and subtracting. If there are several numbers to add or subtract, he gets lost in the arithmetic. She walks Joe down a hallway through a few new areas and then asks him to find his way back. He's able to partially find his way back, but not completely.

I've been with Joe for his evaluations at MGH, and I can see that for whatever reason, he's not showing as much capability as he was a few weeks ago. He seems tired from the testing, although it's not much different from previous tests—maybe a little longer. But he's having his physical, occupational, and cognitive-communication (speech) testing done one after the other, whereas before, they were conducted on different days. The testing takes about an hour and a half, after which she recommends Joe have all three types of therapy twice a week starting next week. She suggests I call on Monday to set up appointments. I'm not surprised by her recommendations, but I'm worried about Joe's responsiveness to the tests.

As we leave the facility, I can't help comparing it to MGH. Clearly, it's well supplied with equipment and multiple areas to work with many patients. It's an impressive-looking institute. The tests today were very thorough, and the diagnosis isn't really a surprise. But what I do find surprising was the discussion about Joe's illness and that when I asked about the staff's experience working with patients with glioblastoma, the response was somewhat vague. Clearly they have experience with many types of brain-related trauma and with common types of brain tumors, but glioma is a unique condition. I'm not sure how much experience the staff has with gliomas and with patients who've had brain radiation. We want the best care Joe can have, and this hospital is highly recommended, so we decide to continue. The drive home is long and tiring for Joe, and he sleeps much of the way home. We have a late dinner, and then Joe goes to bed early.

◆

Much has happened over the past week, and Joe and I compare our thoughts over breakfast Saturday morning. In other words, I do a lot of the talking and Joe weighs in in his indirect manner. Joe sits at the dining table with the *Wall Street Journal* in front of him, front page up, while I prepare breakfast. Scrambled eggs, toast, bacon, and fruit are Joe's favorites, while I prefer oatmeal and fruit. As we eat breakfast, I look down the table at Joe. He appears rested after the evaluation yesterday, so I ask him what he thought about it. He continues to look at the newspaper as he answers.

"It was a long drive to get there, and it was tiring," he says. "I feel better from the infusion on Wednesday, but think I'm feeling the radiation."

My chest tightens at his answer as I think about his fatigue. I suppose it confirms what I suspected might be happening, but to hear Joe acknowledge it is something else.

He looks at me and says, “Bennett is coming over this afternoon. I haven’t seen him since I had surgery. I wonder what’s going on with him and Steff.”

“Yes, and Jim and Allison will be here early evening for a couple of days,” I reply. “Do you want to walk this morning before Bennett comes over?” So we decide to walk around the neighborhood in an hour.

I tell Joe that while Bennett is here, I plan to meet with a local real estate agent. The agent (whom I’ll call “L”) has sold many homes in our neighborhood, and I want to talk to her about listing our home. I think we may be better off trying to sell it as a three-bedroom house, which means we’ll need to modify our den. I mention it to Joe, and he nods. It’s not a big project, but it’ll need a permit and licensed contractor to complete.

After I clean up our breakfast dishes, Joe and I put on our coats and hats and head out for our walk. Joe’s favorite coat is a cobalt blue windbreaker my mother and father gave to him for Christmas several years ago. His hat is a black wool knit lumberjack pull-on. He chooses a pair of sneakers with deep sole tread from among several pairs lined up near our front door. We step down three steps to our sidewalk, walk to the end of the driveway and cross the street to the sidewalk surrounding the housing development green.

As we walk past Ray and Lynette’s front yard, Ray sees us and walks over to us, asking us how we’re doing. We answer with the usual pleasantries and mention that we’re moving to Florida. I explain that we want to have the house ready to sell by the middle of June, hoping to attract a buyer that wants to move during the summer, and that we’re thinking of converting our den to a third bedroom. Ray and Lynette are moving in July and recently found a buyer for their home.

We compare our approaches, and Ray gives us advice based on what he learned selling his home. Ray knows the health issue with Joe and that we're dealing with a lot. He's very helpful sharing his home selling experience, and we appreciate his insight.

After lunch, Bennett arrives. Neither of us has seen him in several months, and I wonder what he'll think when he sees Joe. They've texted about University of Tennessee sports, golf, and Joe's general condition. But seeing Joe is something altogether different. It's so important that Joe surround himself with people he cares about. And Bennett, whom he's known since their freshman year in college, is in this category.

"Ben, so good to see you," Joe says as he invites Bennett in and they shake hands. Joe looks over Bennett's shoulder and sees a gold convertible sports car.

"Whoa, nice ride," he says. "Lynn, take a look at this!" He turns back to Bennett and tells him, "I test-drove this model a year or so ago, and it was too rich for me. But what a good choice and a fine automobile. How long have you had it?"

Bennett agrees it's a sweet ride and says he picked it up about a week ago, then adds, "You know, I kind of forgot how to get here—it's been a while since I've been over."

They both laugh and take seats in the TV area—Joe in the grog chair and Bennett on the sofa. Bennett asks Joe how he's doing and what he's been up to. Joe tells him about living in Boston, and when he brings up the MGH treatments, he asks me to get his radiation mask to show to Bennett. I give Joe the mask and he places it over his face, and jokes that it's his "Hannibal Lecter look—great for next Halloween." Bennett laughs, and Joe hands him the radiation mask so he can feel the texture of the mesh. Joe doesn't elaborate much on his current treatment other than to comment that he's continuing with physical therapy.

Joe tells Bennett about our plan to move to Florida, hopefully by the end of the summer. Bennett talks about how he and Steff sold their home and are enjoying living in their new rental condominium in downtown Hartford. Joe has seen it, but I haven't, so Bennett describes it a little. They talk about their children for a bit before they decide to watch a University of Tennessee Orange and White spring football game on TV. That makes it easy for me to excuse myself to see the real estate agent.

L's office is in our housing development's unfinished clubhouse, which is currently being used as a sales office. She's unpacking her tote bag when I walk in, and she looks up at me and smiles.

"Hey, Lynn, how's it going?" she asks.

"As good as can be expected," I reply "Joe has a friend visiting, so I thought I'd come by and talk to you for a minute. Do you have some time?"

"Yes, I have a few minutes before my appointment. What's up?" she says.

L knows about Joe's illness, so I tell her we want to sell our house and move to Florida. I ask her if she'd consider taking our listing as long as it won't be a conflict of interest for her, since she helps sell new homes for the development builder. She says that she doesn't work directly for the builder so she doesn't think there's a conflict and would be glad to list the house for us. She says she'll prepare a contract and bring it to us by the middle of next week. We discuss the terms, and she agrees that putting the house on the market in late May or early June is a good idea to work with buyers that want to move into a new school district over the summer. She also recommends that we convert the house to a three-bedroom if we can.

Now we have a direction to work toward, and I know we have six weeks to get the home ready for prospective buyers to view. The house is in good shape other than the things I have to sort through that have "collected" in the unfinished side of the basement. Since we have a home in Florida that's already furnished, much of what we have will go to family or friends or will be sold. The house will be shown with furniture, and clearing out the basement is the second priority to turning the den into a bedroom. I thank her and walk back to our house.

I arrive at the house as Bennett is telling Joe that he needs to leave and meet Steff. Joe walks him to the door and then steps outside to "direct" Bennett as he backs his car out of the driveway. They wave at each other; then Joe and I go back inside. Joe retires to the sunroom and stretches out on the sofa, where the cats quickly join him—Rascal at his side and Simba at his feet. Joe enjoys the late-afternoon sun on his face and closes his eyes. He's fast asleep in seconds.

There's a soft knock on the front door, and I open it to see Ray on the doorstep. He asks how Joe is doing, and I tell him he's asleep in the sunroom. He motions me to step outside for a minute so we don't disturb Joe.

Ray tells me that he's been talking things over with Lynette and he thinks he has some free time now that their house is under contract. He's a licensed electrician and knows a lot about home construction. A few years ago, he converted a room over his garage into a third bedroom. He offers to convert our den to a third bedroom. Ray explains that he'd do the electrical work and finishing, such as taping the drywall and painting, and his friend Al would be the contractor and would be responsible for the framing and drywall. I'm so touched that he'd make such an offer, knowing how hard it would be for me to find a contractor I could trust to do the work. I try not to cry, because I know how much it would embarrass Ray–not to mention myself. I manage to hold it together, and I nod that I would like the help. He agrees to draw up a proposal itemizing the work, cost, and schedule. He tells me he thinks the job can be complete in three weeks or so, once the permit is approved by the city. After all, we already have a partial wall in place; we only need to close the existing six-foot opening and add a door.

Ray says he'll bring me the proposal in a day or two, and if I agree, he'll start. I can't thank him enough, and he leaves quickly—I think he's a little embarrassed by my reaction. I close the front door after he leaves, and I lean back against the wall. What a wonderful thing for Ray to offer us! I never know who will come to our aid, and so unexpectedly. I silently thank God for the help.

At around 7 p.m., Jim and Allison arrive from Ashburn, Virginia, about six hours away. We all greet one another before I show them to the room they'll be staying in. Joe stays downstairs while we complete the lodging logistics, then we return downstairs to discuss dinner plans. We decide to pick dinner up from a local Chinese restaurant. Jim stays with Joe while Allison and I go to pick up the food. It takes fifteen minutes to drive to the restaurant, and our food is ready when we arrive. Along the drive, Allison and I discuss Joe's condition, Allison's and Jim's jobs, and their lifestyle in Ashburn. I fill her in on Joe's diagnosis, telling her how serious it is. Allison and Jim understand and want to see Joe and help if they can. Just having them visit is such a help to us. They're very easy guests to have in the house—thoughtful, observant, and eager to assist with almost anything that needs to be done. When we get home with the food, we set up the dining room table and then enjoy dinner once everyone is seated.

When Joe and his brother are together it's as if they speak a language only the two of them know. Their mannerisms, hand gestures, slow smiles, dark-brown eyes that express delight in humorous surprises—all are very similar. They both remember many jokes and situations they shared when they were growing up and make half-sentence references that they both understand. Allison and I follow along as best we can, interrupting on occasion with "What does that mean?" There are stories about an unfinished basement where they could draw on the walls, and where their mother would play the piano in the basement while they sang and danced. Now, Jim is an accomplished pianist and guitar player who sings with a light baritone voice, whereas Joe used to play the piano and trombone but didn't keep up with it.

They recite lines from *Star Trek* and compare dexterity by doing the iconic "live long and prosper" hand gesture. Joe wiggles his ears, and Jim laments that he never could do it like Joe could. They compare early golf rounds with their father and joke about the "rules" for caddies. It's a fun dinner, and I see how much Joe is enjoying himself. It's over much too soon, as it's clear Joe is fighting to stay and extend the fun for as long as he can even though he's getting tired. We all go to bed at around 10 p.m., readying ourselves for our time together over the next couple of days.

◆

I go to an early Mass the next morning while the others sleep. It's now Joe's routine to rest until 8:30 a.m., so I can leave and return to him sleeping. When Greg had surgery in 2014, my father lent me a rosary that his grandmother had passed on to him. He later gave it to me keep, and I constantly use it now as I pray that Joe will recover. Even with Joe's diagnosis, I still hope for a turnaround. Mass provides me solace, a place to think and gain perspective. I also pray to accept what the future holds and to have the strength to deal with it.

When I get back home, Jim is sitting at the dining room table on his laptop. I make coffee and breakfast, knowing Joe will be awake soon. Meanwhile, Jim casually asks me questions about how Joe is really doing. I don't hold anything back, and I explain that the clinical trial* is risky in that it's only phase II, but we know that other treatments are less effective. So, this is the best treatment we know about, and we hope it will be beneficial. I ask Jim what he observes about Joe, and he says he can see Joe is tired. He offers to help me with anything he can, especially knowing we're preparing to move. I decide to take him up on his offer, and I make a short list of things he can help with. Joe follows his usual routine and joins us for breakfast before he takes a shower unassisted, then reads the newspaper in the sunroom. Jim keeps him company and they settle into a comfortable camaraderie.

Midday, we drive to Nevers Park, where Joe and I take a slow, comfortable stroll while Jim and Allison take an extended walk. We meet at benches overlooking a local soccer match between middle school children. It's a sunny, cloudless day, unusually warm in the low 70s with a little breeze. We shed our windbreakers as we sit and watch the soccer match, enjoying the children in their excitement over each ball pass and finally when a goal is scored. To see youths with such promising futures ahead is a happy occasion, but the contrast to Joe's circumstances dampens my thoughts. Fortunately, having Jim and Allison with us is a boost to my spirits. Joe and I talk about the many cross-country meets we watched at the park when Greg was in high school. He was a team captain his senior year and so enjoyed the workout and the team competition. The park holds many good memories for us.

We have a relaxed afternoon, with Joe snoozing in the sunroom and Jim helping me move heavy boxes, large plastic storage containers, and an old sofa in the basement. To my amazement, Jim is able to move the sofa out of the basement to the front lawn area, where I'll arrange for the city to pick up as bulky waste. When Joe wakes up, we describe the progress and we start joking about what our neighbors will think about the couch on the side of the road. We start talking about homes we've driven by over the years where junk is left unattended for months, even years, and we decide we should take a picture of our "junkyard" with us sitting on the couch. We file out of the house, and I take a picture of Joe, Jim, and Allison relaxing on the sofa as if they're ready to watch a TV show. We laugh as neighbors drive past and crane their necks, staring at us. We're sure they think the couch is going to be a permanent fixture.

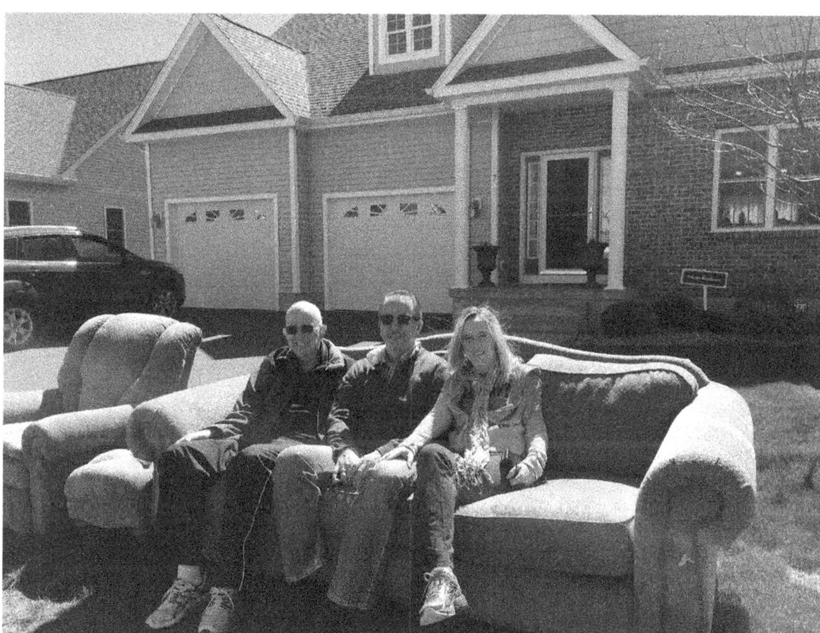

For dinner, Allison prepares the meal kit she brought from Ashburn, purchased from a meal delivery service. It's a very nice recipe, and the ingredients are all very fresh. We enjoy the food and companionship before we enjoy leisurely watching TV in the TV room. We're catching up on season 5 of *Game of Thrones*, knowing season 6 will be airing soon. We watch the episode when Cersei is marched through the city of King's Landing to endure a walk of shame. We all stare at the TV, our attention totally captured. Joe is in the grog chair, and I'm on the couch next to him. I look over at him and see tears running down his face, so I crouch next to him and ask him what's wrong.

"This show is so mean!" he whispers back.

I'm totally surprised. I mean, Joe watched some really graphically violent shows over the years, and I've never seen him have an emotional response like this. When the show is over, I continue to wonder about his reaction. The four of us talk for a while about shows we've watched, and then we retire for the evening. When Joe and I are in bed, I ask him about his reaction to the show. He again says it was so very mean and unnecessary. Okay, so something new is happening with Joe that I need to pay attention to.

Monday is more or less a repeat of Sunday, minus church. We go for a walk, but instead of the park, we go to a nearby apartment complex that has a walking trail around the perimeter. It's closer to our home than the park is, and it provides variety to our daily walk. Jim helps me with window screens in the afternoon, and then we play a game of cards after dinner. My sister Peggy sent me a huge, oversized deck of cards for Christmas one year. I've never opened them, but I decide to use them tonight. It takes us some time to decide what to play, but finally we agree on a game called "C" that Joe's occupational therapist at MGH taught us. It's a memory game where each person is dealt four cards and tries to match their cards from the stack of remaining cards. To build your hand, you have to remember what cards have been discarded. It's a game of chance and memory, with lots of talking that distracts everyone from concentrating.

Shuffling the extra-large cards is a contest among us, but none of us are very good at it. Dealing is pretty straightforward, as the cards slide easily across the table when dealt. It's a good game for Joe to practice his short-term memory. He's quiet during the game, clearly concentrating. We repeat the rules a couple of times, and I think he's a little embarrassed that he has trouble remembering them. Joe is competitive in everything he does, and I'm very protective of him, knowing that he wants to win. We play for a couple of hours, a relaxed, slow-paced game among friends. As we put our cards on the table, Jim declares victory with three Jacks. Joe is the last to put his cards on the table, an impish grin on his face. He slowly reveals his hand—four kings, the winning hand! We all laugh at the dramatic way he shows his cards, and then he puts them together like a fan and poses for the winner photo that Jim takes.

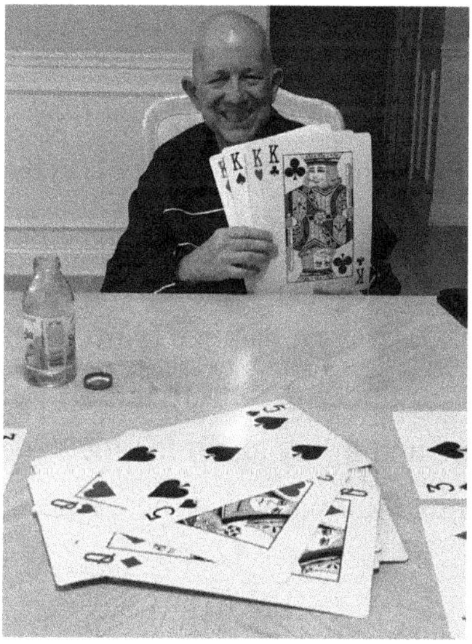

This ends our evening with Jim and Allison, and we all retire to our rooms for the night. Joe is tired from exercising his memory and falls asleep quickly. I'm a little keyed-up from today's events, so I decide to log on to the MGH patient portal* to read the doctor's written report from Joe's last visit. They're usually available a few days after an appointment. Joe continues to be tired, and his short-term memory is sporadic, which causes me to continually worry. Because I understand so little of his illness, I'm constantly looking for more information. I suspect the doctors know much more than they're telling us and are keeping any conjecture to themselves.

Logging in to the portal and finding reports from doctor visits is easy, so I find the radiology report from our latest appointment. They seem to support continuing Joe's treatment, but they also suggest caution. I refuse to acknowledge the possibility that Joe is anything but getting better. I can't imagine a day without him, I'm so desperate for him to recover. I can't ignore what I read, but I also focus on the doctor visit where it was decided that Joe would continue treatment. The report makes the situation grimmer than what I understood from the doctor's appointment. I'm with Joe every day, and I'm watching him carefully. On the one hand, he seems okay; on the other, the fatigue and the issues with short-term memory persist. Even if he stays the way he is now, I still have him with me. We still talk everything over—whether it's about moving, finances, wills, people, or work—just like we always have. He continues to provide sound perspective on any conversation we have, always a balance to my input. I can't imagine a time when it'll stop. So I put my faith in the doctors and their decision to continue treatment, and I pray again for Joe's recovery. I file this report away in my mind, knowing that there's no guarantee for the future—only hope.

◆

Jim and Allison leave Tuesday morning, with Joe "directing" Jim as he backs their car out of our driveway. Their visit was such a boost for us, as we enjoy being with them so much. We're now back to our routine, with daily walks, follow-up exercises, and appointments at the therapy hospital. Word is out that Joe is home, so there are many people who ask to visit. The first is Al, a retired peer and longtime friend of Joe's with a larger-than-life personality. He starts visiting Joe once a week and is a welcome visitor. He talks almost nonstop, expounding on current events, his life as a retiree, and updates about work. Joe finds the visits invigorating yet fatiguing. He jokingly comments that he feels like Al's student, because he listens much more than he talks during these visits. Al is very generous with his time, and he brings books for Joe to read. Both Joe and I greatly appreciate that he visits.

One day, Al brings over a book that's over 1,000 pages long, with fine print. The next day, Joe picks it up and stretches out on the couch in the sunroom to read it. In the meantime, I'm busy sorting boxes that I brought up from the basement in preparation for our move to Florida. At lunchtime, around four hours later, Joe declares that he's finished the book. I'm quite amazed, even though he's always been a fast reader.

"Really?" I say.

"Yes," he replies. "You know I'm a fast reader."

"What was it about?" I ask him.

He tells me little more than the words on the book cover sleeve. Aaah, I think to myself. What's going on? I pick up the book, scan a section, and start to discuss it with him. He waves his hand at me and says he doesn't remember that part. I go to another section and get the same result. After a few more tries, I can see that he hasn't read the book but wants to believe that he has. I don't press him, knowing that he must be trying to convince himself and me that he really read the book as fast as he would've in the past. Except there was never a time when he would've been able to read 1,000 pages in four hours. That's what tipped me off that something wasn't right. I don't want to hurt his dignity or press on the fact that he appears to have read only the book cover—or that he'd read more but retained only the content on the cover. But I think about it and what it may mean about his state of mind and reading retention skills.

It took some coordination with the therapy center to establish successive appointment times for each type of therapy two times a week. It doesn't always work out, so sometimes we have to have three days of appointments in order to meet with each therapy discipline twice weekly. Joe has a different speech therapist and physical therapist for every appointment, though he sometimes has continuity with the occupational therapist. Physical therapy involves various approaches applied with different exercises. Some might focus on flexibility, others on balance, and others on strength or aerobic conditioning. We never know what will be worked on. Sometimes we're given homework, other times no. One thing all the therapists recommend is walking, which we do on days when there are no appointments.

The purpose of the speech therapy is to work with short-term memory. Sometimes Joe is asked to complete puzzles, match number sequences, or answer questions about something he's been asked to read. Other times he uses a large computer screen and works through various layers of electronic tasks by answering computer-generated questions or matching picture and number sequences. The instructions can be difficult to understand, so Joe sometimes struggles with it. The tool has impressive potential, but is not used at each therapy session so it has limited impact on Joe's improvement.

There's some overlap between occupational therapy and speech therapy in that some tasks involve taking apart and putting together various gadgets, an activity Joe excels at consistently. His weakness is in lower-level math, as when he tries to balance a checkbook. He has no trouble filling out checks or adding items to a calendar when he's told when and where to add them. But when he's asked to *remember* an appointment and put it on a calendar, he has difficulty. He's given homework to write down what he does every day. He's also asked to write down his daily pill schedule, but he gets confused about it if I leave it entirely up to him. I purchased a couple of pill boxes and set up a spreadsheet so he could follow a printed timeline, but it doesn't solve the problem. So I took control of that task myself, knowing how important it is for him to take all his medicine exactly as prescribed. Joe is taking only a few medicines—for high cholesterol, high blood pressure, and Crohn's disease*—but even with occupational therapy, it's too much for him to keep track of.

Joe isn't very interested in doing the homework he's asked to do, even knowing he's supposed to bring it with him to each appointment. Between appointments, I work with him to finish the activities, prodding him to completion. He won't do the work if I don't remind him, and I can't understand why. As far as I can tell, he simply isn't excited about doing the homework, so he forgets. I explain over and over that these tasks can help him rebuild brain connections that will strengthen his memory skills, but to little avail. He's more interested in walking or doing some exercises, but the exercises are more of a struggle for him when they were six weeks ago, when he had radiation fatigue. I insist that he do every homework assignment even though it's clear the mental homework is very tiring for him. His handwriting is becoming wobbly, less sure than it ever was. He's right-handed, so his handwriting hasn't typically been affected by his essential tremor, which occurs on his left side. It appears to be an ever-so-slight yet continuing decline in handwriting capability. I tell each of his therapists about Joe's issues with the mental homework and his handwriting, so the occupational therapist spends time working with him on his handwriting. He does some practice exercises that the therapist gives him, and his handwriting stops getting worse over a couple of weeks but doesn't improve.

Joe seems to respond well when he has an established relationship with his therapists. This is difficult to accomplish with the schedule also set up to minimize the number of days we travel to the facility. We're not building the rapport we would like with Joe's speech and physical therapists, which impacts Joe's motivation. He responds so well to those he works with routinely.

◆

The remainder of the month of April and the month of May includes three trips to MGH for infusion treatments; continued physical, occupational, and speech therapy at the facility in Connecticut; and visits from Joe's friends and colleagues. The infusion process remains the same, and we stay with Greg on each trip. We usually don't see Dr. D on infusion visits; instead, we see Nurse N. She's supportive of our plan to move to Florida and travel twice a month from there to Boston for Joe's continued treatment, beginning in October if we sell our home in Connecticut. We're planning a trial trip to Florida after Joe's next MRI, which is scheduled for June 7. We want to assess whether it'll be feasible to fly back and forth to MGH, with a two-week rest period in Florida. We've established a routine around our visits to MGH, and it's been working pretty well considering it takes a day and a half. Joe consistently comments that he feels better after an infusion treatment, usually a day or so after. He appears refreshed and has more energy, but he still has issues with short-term memory.

During this six-week period, there's a great deal of activity in addition to Joe's treatment and therapy. Ray and Al are finishing the conversion of the den into a third bedroom as we prepare to list our house on June 1. The project is going quite well—Al and Ray are on schedule, and they're doing a great job. It involves framing, drywall, electrical work, and hanging and painting a door. It's not a large project, so they usually come over for just two to three hours at a time a couple of times a week. Ray often comes over when we're at one of Joe's appointments, so there's very little work done when we're in the house.

My sisters Peggy and Kathy and my nephew Sean, under Peggy's organization, are coordinating the move of our belongings from one house in Florida to our new home farther north. Both sisters have large SUVs, which they use to transport pictures, glassware, clothes, lamps, bedding, and towels. Sean is responsible for labeling and packing the electronics, and he has the "muscle" for moving large items. Sean also drives Joe's dad's older car to the new home. It's a 1991 Buick LeSabre with gold paint and beige velour seats—a comfortable if not stylish ride.

All three of them work together to spackle and paint holes made by wall hangings and to thoroughly clean the entire house. It's a huge undertaking, and they finish the packing in two days. Peggy coordinates with the moving company I contracted with in December and supervises when they remove the furniture from our home and again when they unload it from the moving van and position it in our new home. Once all our belongings have been moved in, Peggy, Kathy, and Sean arrange them in the appropriate places throughout the house. They also organize the electronics so I can set them up easily when I need to. Peggy also returns our TV modem to the cable company and coordinates a walk-through with our Realtor. I can never repay the kindness the three of them showed by their help. It's incredible that they would do all that and do such a truly excellent job.

After much soul searching, I decide to officially retire, with a final work date of May 15. I've worked in aerospace for 37 years and love the work, but there's nothing as important as Joe. I have no way of knowing how much time he has, and there's nothing more significant than being with him for as long as possible. I've been offered an opportunity to take a long leave from work, with the understanding that I'd return as things take their course. But I can't imagine working without Joe in an area that we've shared throughout our lives. Just the thought of going into buildings that he's been at day in and day out, working with so many people who know him—I'm simply not strong enough to do it. I discuss it with my boss and our HR department and let them know my decision.

Greg comes to Connecticut almost every weekend so he can see us as much as possible. One Sunday morning when he's home, I take the opportunity to drive to work so I can organize my files for my successor and remove my personal items. I'm almost certain that no one will be in the office area on a Sunday morning, so I'll have privacy, knowing it will be emotional for me. My retirement hasn't been announced and I don't want to create any controversy or angst within the workforce while succession planning is determined. I take my usual route to work, following I-84W. Traffic is light, and the weather clear but slightly cloudy with the temperature in the low 50s.

As I enter the main campus, my mind is flooded with so many memories, and I feel temporary remorse for not accepting the offer to return at a later date. I also have many memories of the many, many times I would see Joe at work—walking through a hallway, on the shop floor, in the cafeteria, in the museum, or in the lab. As I pass each building, there's something else to remind me of Joe. There's a part of Joe and me left here, through the many years of work. I park my car and walk to my office using a walkway that Joe wouldn't have taken to access his work space. I take the elevator, exit left, and enter my office.

Thank goodness I remembered where I kept my office key, since I haven't been here in a couple of months as I was accessing work remotely. I sit at my desk for what is likely the last time, then begin opening my desk drawers to organize information and sort through my personal belongings. As I expected, I become emotional as I pack up my mementos, pictures, plaques, and airplane models—many going back to the late 70s—that I've kept with me from job to job and from location to location. I electronically organize files so others can access them, and I leave hardcopy files clearly labeled. The process takes longer than I thought it would, but I feel some modicum of closure as I close my office door, locking it behind me.

Joe's friends and colleagues continue to visit. Joe, the social personality he is, welcomes the visits. But he's also apprehensive, and he tells me he's embarrassed that he looks somewhat different and that he's so careful walking, standing up, and sitting down. He asks me if it's noticeable that conversations are slower because he sometimes takes a while to think about his answer before he speaks.

"I don't want people to see me as sick or incapacitated," he says. And I don't want anyone feeling sorry for me."

I try to reassure him by telling him that the people coming to see him are friends who wish him well and want him to be better as soon as possible.

"It's not like you don't understand them, can't hear, or can't see. You're recovering from a major surgery and radiation treatment, and they know how serious that is," I say. "They don't feel sorry for you, Joe; they're just sorry you have this illness. There's a big difference.

I remind him that his colleagues Jean, Mike, and Chris will be bringing pizza on Saturday and really want to spend time with him.

"I hope you won't worry about it," I add. "You're so much yourself that they'll be relieved."

Joe usually isn't so direct about his feelings, so the conversation surprises me a bit. He really is worried, or he wouldn't have brought it up. Every chance I get, I compliment on him what he's doing so he'll feel less self-conscious.

Jean, Mike, and Chris arrive at around 11:30 a.m., carrying boxes of pizza. It's from Giovanni's Brick Oven Pizzeria, which was the favorite lunch location for Joe and Mike.

Joe walks from the sunroom to the front door to welcome his friends. "So good to see you, come on in!" he says.

Jean also brings a plastic container with some homemade brownies. We decide to set the pizza on the dining room table and put the baked goods on the kitchen island.

Jean gives Joe a hug. "Joe, I'm so glad to see you," she says. "We all miss you in the office. It's not the same without you there."

"It's hard to believe, but I think I miss being there!" Joe replies with a smile, and they all chuckle.

Joe and his visitors take seats in the dining room—Joe at the head of the table, Chris opposite him. I get plates from the kitchen cabinet and put them on the table. They talk about various projects and updates on people they know. Chris asks if it's okay if a couple of people contact him with questions, and Joe nods his agreement.

Mike starts describing the office environment. They also discuss plans to relocate the department to another building, though they'll be moving to a staging area first. Mike says he's packed up Joe's desk for the move and asks him if there are personal items he'd like to have from his office. Joe says he'd like to have the personal photographs from his office, and they talk about the things Joe had in his office that people enjoyed stopping by to "use." One was a billiard ball that would "predict the future" by answering the user's yes/no questions, and they joke about how they used to consult it for important technical decisions. They also joke about how often Mike would stop into Joe's office under the pretense of discussing work, only to practice solving the "golf ball in the water globe" brain teaser.

"It's no wonder you're so good at it—you were always practicing!" Joe says. "I, on the other hand, always had too much work to practice!"

Then Mike says he came across something unusual when he was packing up Joe's desk.

"Way in the back of one of your desk drawers, I found a stack of business cards that makes me think I don't know you as well as I thought," he jokes "Have you had a second career on the side that we should know about?"

Joe looks puzzled and shrugs his shoulders.

"Maybe, but I'll never tell," he smiles. "What did you find?"

Mike reaches into his pocket and slides something across the table to him. I'm listening from the kitchen, wondering what they're talking about, and I hear Joe laugh when he sees it.

"Hey, Lynn, take a look at this!" he calls to me in the kitchen.

I join the group and lean over Joe's shoulder, and I laugh too when I see what it is: a light-gray business card printed with the initials "GJG," a large imprint of red lips, and Joe's name and address from 1980. Joe tells the story of the card.

> "I leave work at 4 p.m., I'm wearing slacks, a long-sleeve button-down shirt, and a tie. I am driving the two-lane road into the small city of Palm Beach Gardens, turning east on PGA Boulevard. I turn south on Military Trail and make a left turn into Tanglewood Plaza. I don't want to be late for my haircut, because my curly hair needs some containment. I'm starting to show some gray hair, but what can I do? Must be hereditary, since the same happened to my mother.
>
> Anyway, my 1972 Pontiac Grand Prix, which I fondly named "The Nimitz," had a limited turning radius and was very long, so it was a struggle to park it. When I'm finally parked, I run to the hair salon and take a seat, waiting for my turn. My usual stylist isn't working today, so I don't know who'll be cutting my hair. I hear my name called, and I look up to be greeted by a woman in her late 20s named Shelly. When I stand up, I notice I'm much taller than Shelly, which makes me feel lanky compared to her. She sits me in the last of four chairs, and I notice a colleague in the second chair as I walk by. We nod at

each other in acknowledgment. Shelly stands behind me and stares at my face in the mirror.

"Oh my God, you look so much like him, I can't believe it!" she exclaims loudly. "Well, this is my lucky day. The chance to cut hair like his—I mean, who would've thought it? You even walk like he does and are dressed like he was in the movie!"

She has a very loud voice, and my colleague looks over to see what's happening. I have no idea what she's talking about, but she continues to ramble. "I know exactly how to cut your hair, so leave everything to me. She says. "Oooh, that was the best movie I've ever seen. Do you believe that ending? Sooooo romantic. Have you seen it? What do you think?"

I shrug and ask her what movie she's talking about.

"*American Gigolo,* of course!" she says. "Richard Gere—oh, he was so great in the movie. And you look so much like him, I can't get over it!"

The whole time she cuts my hair, she talks about the movie. Talk about a spoiler alert. Good thing I wasn't planning to see the movie. Why would I need to after this haircut? She finishes with my hair, and I sheepishly walk past my colleague, raising my hand in a gesture that says, "What can you do?"

The next morning, I settle into my chair at my drawing board and notice a few people congregated in my boss's office. They're chuckling, and a couple of times, someone turns to look at me. My phone rings, and my boss calls me to his office. As I walk up to his desk, I ignore the stares of my colleagues in his office. My boss asks me to take a seat.

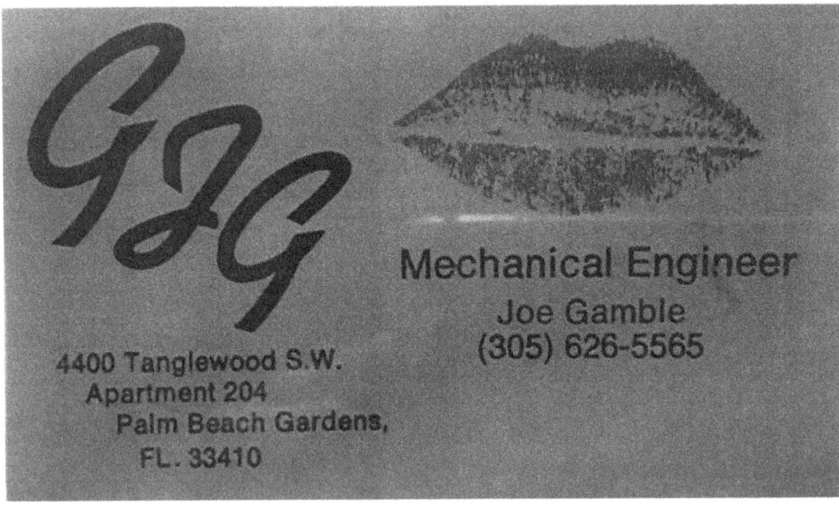

He says, “Joe, I understand that we’re honored to have you with us. We had no idea that you were such a celebrity. Tells us, what’s it like?”

I look around at all the faces looking back at me, trying to figure out what’s going on, and then I ask, “Well, I guess you mean my latest design? You liked it?”

He says, “Well, if you mean designs on you, maybe that’s what this is about. When did you start your second career? Is it acting or some other field? You been hanging around the Palm Beach hotels lately?”

I tell him I don’t understand, and he says, “Well, Paul here tells an interesting story about your haircut yesterday. Seems like you have an admirer. And an interested first client in case you start another profession. So we’d like to present you with a business card in case you need it.”

My boss hands me a box of the business cards you found in my desk and tells me, “The GJG stands for ‘Gigolo Joe Gambill,’ and the lips are for—well, isn’t it obvious?”

They all hoot with laughter at the expression on my face, and they clap each other on the back and say, "Go get 'em, Joe! I guess you won't need a raise this year, with all the extra money you'll be making!" And on and on. For months, whenever I went into a conference room and someone who was there that day was in the room, they'd comment on my hair or ask me how my second job was going. It was all in good fun, and it really was a good joke on me. So I've moved these cards to different offices with me since 1980 as a reminder.

Jean, Mike, and Chris laugh about the story as the card is passed around. Their visit with Joe is over much too soon, and we're sorry when they leave—it's been a huge boost to him. They went to a lot of trouble bringing pizza and Jean's brownies, and we both really appreciated their efforts. Joe stretches out in the sunroom for an afternoon nap. The visit was good for him, but it was also tiring.

◆

On Mother's Day, May 8, we wake up to a day that's a little bit cloudy with temperatures in the mid 50s, expected to reach mid 60s with sun later. Greg is planning to stop by in the early afternoon on his way back from New York, where he spent the weekend visiting friends. Both Joe and I are worried about the strain of Joe's illness on him, and we encourage him to bring his friends over and to visit his friends regularly. We believe that any normalcy he can have in his life now is important. I follow my usual Sunday routine, attending early Mass while Joe sleeps and then helping Joe with his shower, dressing, and breakfast. While we wait for Greg to arrive so we can take Joe's daily walk together, Joe reads the paper on his tablet computer and I bring a box from the basement to sort. I'm avoiding boxes of pictures at this point, so I sort through seasonal clothes we've stored in the basement.

Greg arrives at around 1 p.m., after we finish lunch. He hands me a package and wishes me a happy Mother's Day. It feels soft through the wrapping paper, and I have no idea what it is. With Joe and Greg watching, I unwrap the present. It's a round pillow, the same color as our "peep pillow," with a happy face on it. I look up at Greg and laugh.

"Mom I know how you've been missing the peep pillow, and I was worried about you," he tells me. "So, I brought you a replacement. Hope you like it!"

I throw the pillow at him and joke, "I'll find some use for it. Thanks, so very thoughtful of you!" Joe and Greg laugh while I decorate the sunroom sofa with it.

The three of us go to Nevers Park for a walk. Joe and Greg walk side by side, and I lag behind a little. Joe occasionally throws Greg a soft shoulder punch. Greg is very careful to let Joe set the pace and helps straighten him out when he starts to shift to the left—an issue that seems to be becoming more pronounced each day. It's not a sharp veer to the left, but it's gradual enough that Joe doesn't realize it's happening. When Joe and I walk alone, he gets a little frustrated with me if I remind him to focus on walking in a straight line. With Greg, he cheerfully accepts the input to walk straight and focuses. But I do understand that when you're a daily caregiver and the patient is your husband, your input isn't always appreciated. After our walk, we go to the Dairy Delight to get ice cream, which Joe loves. We sit outside people watching and watching cars drive down Route 5, enjoying the afternoon and being together.

I hired Greg's friend Colin to help me clear our accumulated possessions out of the basement. On weekends, Greg and Colin are helping me find homes for many useable items we won't be taking with us. We started in April, and it's been slow going. I'm ashamed at how much we've accumulated in our unfinished section of basement—albums, old stereo equipment, unused furniture, textbooks from college days, boxes of clothing we haven't used in years, and more. The items are somewhat organized, but I still need to look each one over and decide whether to throw it out, donate it, or sell it.

There are also crates of photos that I plan to sort, but not until I feel emotionally strong enough, because each memory brings me to tears. I watch our lives pass by over the years through the many pictures I look at. I can't accept that it's coming to a close—I simply won't believe it. I show Joe several of the pictures, and we laugh about the many good times we've had together. I constantly fluctuate emotionally from optimism to fear to overwhelmed. My emotions are so raw, I know I'm not thinking straight. It helps me if I focus on something I can do, like getting the house ready to sell as I know I can't heal Joe. Why isn't there more information about his disease? I agonize over it every day.

Joe's immunotherapy treatments continue to be successful: his bloodwork before the treatment and his vital signs during it are within the normal expected ranges. He still feels better after each treatment, and the fatigue from the radiation therapy has been getting less severe. Joe's therapy sessions at the facility in Connecticut continue to have little consistency from visit to visit, and his short-term memory has improved only slightly. He's physically weaker than he was in Boston, but I'm not sure why. He's doing his exercises with my encouragement, and he's walking, although slowly. I'm concerned that he's been having more of a problem walking in a straight line, but it's a very gradual change, so I'm hopeful it will improve. He's able to take supervised showers, being careful about balance issues, and he gets dressed with assistance. His essential tremor is a little more pronounced than it was a couple of months ago, though he can feed himself and cut up his own food. His speech hasn't changed, although his voice is a little quieter than before.

Near the end of May, Joe's sister Jane and her husband Jim visit us for a long weekend. Jim is handy in the kitchen and cooks a delicious dinner one night, which is such a help to me. We take a couple of walks all together and enjoy the beautiful New England spring season, with magenta azaleas and pink flowering dogwood trees in full bloom. Jim and Jane ask many questions about Joe's condition and do their best to be optimistic about the diagnosis. We each have our own coping mechanisms for dealing with a family member's terminal illness. Joe is fortunate to have siblings who care so much for him.

The weekend after Jane and Jim leave, Greg visits for a special weekend: we're celebrating Joe's 59th birthday on Saturday. It's our family birthday tradition that the day be devoted to the person being celebrated. It starts with breakfast, followed by activities and dinner of the honoree's choice. Joe requests chocolate chip pancakes, eggs, bacon, fruit, and toast for breakfast, which we eat at the dining room table. Greg and Joe lounge in the sunroom for a bit before Joe opens his presents with the "help" of the kitties. One of Greg's presents to Joe is a package of practice golf balls, so we immediately head to the back yard. I get Joe's 7-iron for him so he can try to hit the ball. It's the first time he's had a golf club in his hand since his surgery, and Greg and I watch closely. Joe is being very cautious, and he keeps his backswing to a quarter swing. He manages without incident, and Greg joins him for a short competition. It's hard to know who the winner is on this blustery day, but it doesn't matter: what's most important is that Joe has a golf club in his hand again.

The next day, Joe wants to go to the Willowbrook driving range. His success with the practice balls was exciting, and he wants to try to hit a few balls at the range. Once again, Joe is cautious and stays with quarter swings. His contact with the ball is nowhere ncar his standard of play, but he persists for close to fifteen minutes before he decides to use the practice putting green. Joe and Greg begin a putting competition, but Joe stops shortly after starting. He and I sit in chairs facing the practice range while Greg continues hitting golf balls. He has a beautiful golf swing, and although he doesn't practice much, he's hitting the ball well. Joe watches him proudly.

"That's my boy—a chip off the old block!" he says.

Joe is content to watch, and I ask him how he's feeling.

"Not bad, but it's frustrating for me not to be able to hit the ball very well," he responds. "I'm not ready to take a full backswing. I can feel the shift in balance even with a quarter swing, and I'm afraid I might fall. I love to play golf, but not like this. Even my putting was off.

"I do like watching Greg practice, though," he adds. "Too bad he doesn't play more often."

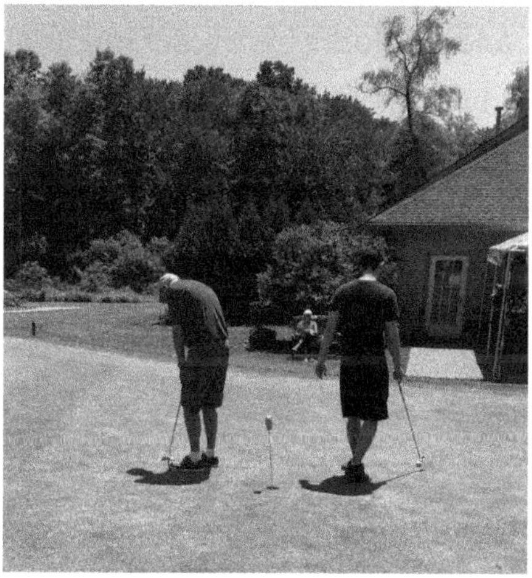

◆

Joe's second post-radiation MRI is scheduled for June 7. We follow our now-typical process for an MRI without event. We take a morning walk around the neighborhood to make sure we get some exercise before we travel to Boston. Driving requires a lot of concentration because of the heavy truck traffic into Boston. We drive to Greg's apartment and stay there for a couple of hours, which gives Joe a chance to rest a little before we go to the hospital for his MRI at 5 p.m.

We know the way to MGH, but since we don't usually go there from Greg's apartment during the late-afternoon rush hour, we give ourselves extra time to allow for traffic. It's only a 2-mile drive, but it takes about 50 minutes to get to the parking garage near the main entrance. Joe wants to walk with me from the garage to the entrance, but he agrees to use a wheelchair from the entrance to the MRI area. I am so thankful that Joe has regained enough strength to walk unaided. I know it makes him feel so much more in control and independent. We're familiar with both the location and the routine of the MRI process, and everything goes smoothly.

As we drive back to Greg's apartment afterward, the motion of the car seems to relax Joe, and he closes his eyes. Greg is at his apartment when we arrive, and he helps walk Joe up the sidewalk, into the elevator, and down the corridor to the apartment. We eat the prepared dinner I brought from home, and then Joe goes to bed early. With the door to the bedroom open, I can see and hear him from the TV room. He doesn't get up once during the night, which isn't typical for him—he usually needs to go to the bathroom at least once a night, and I go with him to make sure he's appropriately balanced.

I'm well rested in the morning, and I help him shower and get dressed. To my surprise, he's still feeling some of the effects of the sedative he had taken for the MRI and is slow moving in general. He's well balanced, thankfully. Putting on his socks and shoes is a challenge, but we manage and then have breakfast.

We drop Greg off at his office on our way to MGH from Greg's Brookline apartment. Every time he leaves, I feel a tug at my heart. It's the natural progression of growing up, and Joe and I were very deliberate in trying to be sure that he would become an independent adult, able to care for himself. But that doesn't mean I don't miss him and selfishly want him to stay with us.

We follow our usual routine, now parking at the Yawkey Center parking garage for Joe's infusion treatments. We go to the 9th floor for Joe's bloodwork, then meet with Dr. D to review the results of Joe's MRI. We're excited about our upcoming trip to Florida on June 10. I have my worries about travel logistics, but that's one of the purposes of this trip: to establish exactly how hard it may be. Nurse N joins us in the patient room and conducts her usual review. She looks at the blood test results and confirms that they're within expected ranges. We tell her about our travel plans, and she wishes us well. Dr. D joins us,

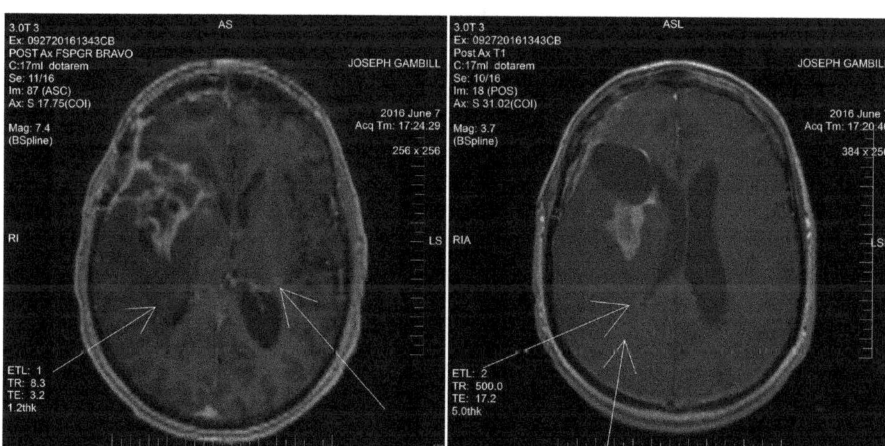

and Joe asks him how he's doing and congratulates him on his recent marriage. Dr. D looks surprised that Joe knows about his wedding (his nurse had told us), but he tells us a little about it and completes his preliminary tests with Joe.

Dr. D swivels in his chair to face the computer in the corner of the room. He logs in and accesses the results of Joe's June 7th MRI. When he finds the image sections he wants to discuss with us, he recommends that Joe proceed with the infusion treatment today. But he adds that the MRI is showing some change that warrants discussion. He explains that the MRI is from three months after the radiation, which may have influenced it slightly. Although Joe's vital signs are stable and his exam doesn't show significant changes, Dr. D says he's concerned that the MRI indicates T2-hyperintensity* and it's possible that the tumor has progressed.

Dr. D recommends that Joe have a short-interval MRI scan in four weeks. He says he'll start Joe on treatment with a steroid called dexamethasone* if he starts showing any new symptoms, like weakness on his left side, headaches, nausea, vomiting, or seizures. He also talks with us about alternate treatment options if the MRI shows tumor progression: other clinical trials, bevacizumab + lomustine, or bevacizumab + temozolomide.* I'm so relieved that Joe is continuing his infusion treatment, but I'm concerned about the MRI results.

Joe and I keep looking at each other while the doctor talks to us. We hear him talking, and we're listening, but we're not processing any of it. We ask about tumor regrowth, but of course there's no definite answer, just the same as before: "no one knows, every case is different, blah, blah, blah." The journey we're on has no answers, just trial treatment—wait and see what happens. I'm ready to scream in anguish.

Joe completes his infusion treatment and we return home—I-90W to I-84W to our exit, like other trips home. Yet somehow, because of the news we've just gotten, it's unlike any of our other trips home. Joe is quiet, resting his head on a pillow in his reclined seat while I drive. I'm usually the one chattering about the drive, the doctor's visit, and the treatment, but not today. I'm trying to absorb what the doctor told us. I'm not accepting the possibilities. I decide I'll wait and read the written doctor's report, then try to come to terms with the information. I have great confidence in the current immunotherapy treatment as Joe always says he feels better after a treatment. How could there be tumor progression if he feels better?* Doesn't make sense to me. We'll see.

◆

Two carry-on suitcases are packed, arrangements for a wheelchair at the airport are made, plans for neighbors to take care of the cats are confirmed, boarding passes are printed… what's left to do? I think we're ready to go. I help Joe down the garage stairs and into the car to ensure he doesn't trip or lose his balance. He can walk, but this trip is uncharted territory for us, so I'm very cautious—I intend to be sure that Joe is safe every step of the way to Florida.

I park the car in the garage of Bradley International Airport and we walk across the enclosed bridge to the airport check-in to pick up a wheelchair. We don't know what today will bring, so Joe is using a wheelchair to help reduce his travel fatigue. An airline employee offers to push the wheelchair while I pull the two carry-on suitcases along. Going through security is fortunately uneventful; we're preapproved for expedited security, which makes the process simpler. Next stop is the gate, where we wait for 40 minutes to board. Joe wants to go to the men's room, so I wheel him there and he walks in unassisted. I wait outside, fretting that he may lose his balance. But he returns without event, and we retrace our steps to the gate area. In all my planning for the trip, I didn't think through how to handle Joe using airport facilities. I'll have to give it more thought, since we're anticipating making the trip to Boston twice a month.

We wait until the boarding process begins, Joe part of the "wheelchair brigade" and me sitting across from him. The wheelchairs are lining up close to the boarding jetway door to the right of the airline attendant check in-desk, where I notice a former colleague and longtime friend of mine. She glances around while she waits, but when she sees me, she quickly looks away. I'm not really surprised at this reaction, but I'm a little disappointed. I don't wave her down, as I've seen this reaction many times since Joe's diagnosis. It's fairly well known that Joe is very seriously ill, and I'm sure my friend has heard, too.

So many people, when faced with a friend's or colleague's life-threatening illness, avoid the circumstance altogether. I'm not sure exactly why, other than that it's a reminder of our shared human condition, which many people may not have come to terms with. Or maybe it's a sad reminder of a friend or relative who has passed, or simply seeing a negative situation that they don't want to be part of. Who knows? I understand that there can be an aversion to a serious illness and recognize that not everyone has the desire or stamina to face the situation head-on. It doesn't mean that they don't care or they're not good people—just that they're limited in that area.

We board the plane without event and fly the three hours non-stop to Palm Beach International Airport. When the plane lands, we wait until all the other passengers have left the plane before we get off so that Joe can access a wheelchair. A wheelchair attendant pushes Joe in his wheelchair to where we can pick up the shuttle to the car rental agency, while I follow behind with our carry-on luggage. We know

PBIA very well as we lived in this area for more than 20 years and then had a second home in the area for an additional nine years. And we so love South Florida. We leave the airport terminal and take in the warm temperature, the light breeze flowing past, and the heavy humid air surrounding us, and we breathe deeply. The blue sky greets us, much brighter than the Connecticut sky we left behind, and we notice the newer construction around us. We're home where we belong.

We thank and tip our wheelchair attendant and then board the shuttle bus once it arrives. Joe has to step up to the bus stairs and then walk up two more stairs to take a seat. He manages with me behind him, ready to help if he needs me. It's another thing I hadn't thought of when I was mentally preparing for the trip. We leave the car rental agency almost seven hours after we left our home to drive to the airport. We drive a little over an hour to our Florida home, making the total travel time close to eight hours. It's a very full day for Joe, and he's handling it quite well. I observe that there's no substitute for the hope and strength that comes when starting to realize a long-awaited dream. Joe has wanted to return to Florida, to live and enjoy the beautiful area, and is so happy we're here, even if only for eight days. I too am happy, but very watchful.

This trip to Florida is the first since Joe was diagnosed and had surgery, radiation treatment, and immunotherapy treatment. I've had such great support from my family long distance, such as my sisters helping me with the sale of one house and moving our belongings to another. The many phone calls, cards, and packages we've received have been such a boost for us over the last six months. My parents, who are in their mid-80s, offered to come to Connecticut to help, but I knew it would be too much for them. My family is planning to arrive in Florida the day after we land and will stay with us until we depart.

It's the first time anyone in my family will see Joe since his diagnosis. Both Joe and I are so looking forward to being with them.

We feel a measure of security by believing we're where we should be. I drive the rental car north on I-95 and Joe suggests we take the PGA Boulevard West exit to Spoto's, one of his favorite restaurants, before we drive the rest of the way home. The area has changed a great deal since we moved to the Northeast, and PGA Boulevard is now a six-lane road with heavy traffic. I park in the area behind the restaurant and we get out of the car. Joe and I walk hand-in-hand into the restaurant, just happy to be together. For an hour or so, while we enjoy a late lunch and time together, it's as if we've gone back in time and left our troubles behind.

After lunch, I drive farther north, taking in the surrounding countryside while paying attention to my driving. Joe talks much of the way, commenting on the changes as we move along, noting new landmarks and buildings. He talks about the new house and is happy about the location, although it's a longer drive from the airport. I exit the interstate, turn west, and drive to our new home. I use the garage door opener and Joe makes his comments about Weather Davenport when I pull in. I laugh and lightly punch his left shoulder after I turn the car off.

I walk around to Joe's side of the car to help him if he needs me to. Together we open the door and walk into the house. We smell the cured concrete, new paint, and tile as we walk through the house. The main living area isn't yet furnished, but the remainder of the rooms are filled with furniture from our home farther south. I had given Peggy sketches of each room to show her where I'd like the furniture, and she did a truly magnificent job with it. There's frozen food in the freezer and bottled water and beverages in the pantry, so I can wait until morning to go to the grocery store. Joe and I walk around from room to room, inspecting the house together, hugging each other with delight. I can never repay my sisters and nephew for their kindness and competence in helping us with the houses. We've arrived at the home where we'll live out our retirement together.

◆

The next morning, Peggy, Sean, and her husband Mike come to visit us. When Peggy arrives at around 10 a.m., I open the front door and greet her with a hug. I'm so happy to see her and so thankful for all she's done for us. Joe walks to the front door to greet her. I can't read her expression as she sees Joe for the first time since his illness, but she walks over to him and gives him a hug.

"Joe, so good to see you," she says. "How are you feeling?"

Joe smiles and says, "I'm feeling pretty good, so glad to be in Florida!"

They walk together into the TV area, and they each take a seat. Our kitchen overlooks the TV area, which is furnished with a loveseat, a sofa, and a recliner. A dinette table and four chairs are also within view of the kitchen. Peggy sits on the loveseat and Joe takes a seat on the sofa. Peggy asks Joe about the trip from Connecticut. "It was a long day, but bearable," he says. They compare notes about the treatments for Joe's brain tumor and Mike's throat cancer. They also discuss current TV shows they've both watched and laugh about various scenes and series endings.

Peggy is talking to Joe as if nothing has happened to him and as if she sees no change. She tells me later that she's determined not to let her thoughts show in what she says or does because she doesn't want Joe to think she pities him. All the while they're talking, she's thinking to herself that he looks better than she expected and seems very lucid.

She's encouraged that he's been helping her convert from Spanish to English on her smartphone, as he's always been skilled at anything electronic. But she also notices that the way he moves is more deliberate, as if he's thinking about his movements instead of quickly reacting, and that his posture seems more stooped than before. She tells me she didn't expect to see so much of a physical change and expected more mental changes.

I greet Mike and Sean at the front door at around 11 a.m. There's room for everyone in the TV room, and we talk about our trip to our new home, including the weather, the traffic, and the route to get here. At lunchtime, we decide to go eat at a local restaurant called the West End Grill, which Peggy tried when she was moving things into the house. We ride together in Peggy's large red SUV. The change in Joe is more noticeable when he gets in and out of the SUV, walks into the restaurant, and navigates to sit in the restaurant. He moves more slowly and has some difficulty using his leg muscles to sit and stand. I suppose I'm used to it, but I can see that my family notices.

After lunch, we watch TV until it's time to eat the food we ordered for dinner. Joe and Mike talk about previous golf outings and joke about my father's golf setup. He's renowned to be a slower golfer, although he claims to play "ready golf." Sean does a pretty good imitation of the setup, including the many foot changes, grip changes, and "butt waggle." Everyone hoots at the imitations and adds their input. It's all in good fun, and my father would laugh about it if he were here, although we would tone it down a bit.

Joe is enjoying the company of family, although he's clearly tired by the end of the day. It's been a good day and he rests very well, getting up only once during the night. I follow him into the bathroom to be sure he doesn't fall. He's steady on his feet, but I'm concerned he might fall in the middle of the night when it's dark and he's in an unfamiliar setting. He wears nonslip socks every night to help prevent him from slipping.

The next morning over breakfast, Joe and Mike talk about sports, comparing teams and players they've followed over the years. Joe has always had a great memory for sports and player stats, often quoting statements from players or reciting events from many years ago. He follows the Southeastern Conference (SEC) of college football, and he's a big fan of the St. Louis Cardinals Major League Baseball team. Mike was an offensive tackle for Florida State University from 1977 to 1981 and is very knowledgeable about football players, events, and stats. He and Joe always love to compare trivia knowledge, and it appears that this morning is no different.

They also spend time discussing their respective cancer treatments, and they have much to share as they've both been through very serious illnesses. It's the first time Joe has been able to talk to another cancer patient at length about his treatment. There are some similarities between their radiation treatments, and discussing the radiation mask and radiation table with someone who has experienced very similar physical and emotional feelings is truly bonding. What these two have endured is beyond my imagination. I couldn't have survived, yet they both have and are talking freely about it.

When Mike and Sean leave that afternoon, Mike looks in Joe's eyes and says, "Hang in there, Joe. I know what you're going through. Take it a day at a time and call me anytime you want to talk about how things are going. I'm thinking about you and wishing you well." They shake hands as a final gesture as Mike turns to leave. Joe, Peggy, and I walk to the driveway and wave as Mike and Sean back out of the driveway and drive off.

My parents are going to arrive in a couple of hours to stay with us for a few days. Peggy is planning to stay the longest, until Thursday. The house has three bedrooms, so I staggered visitors so everyone would have a room to stay in and we wouldn't be too crowded. Also, in consideration of Joe, having many people around is tiring for him as it takes a lot of concentration for him to follow the many conversations and activities. Most people would take it for granted, but for someone with brain cancer, it's not so easy.

When my parents arrive, there are hugs all around as we greet each other. After I help them unpack their car and bring their belongings to their room, we settle in the TV room to catch up. I notice how tired my parents are from the two-hour drive to our house. It's as if they've shrunk since I last saw them six months ago. I'm so glad that I didn't accept their offer to come to Connecticut to help me. They're in their mid 80s, and I can see that it would've been too much for them. I'm worried that the stay with us will be difficult for them, but I know they'll never let on if they're uncomfortable. They both love Joe, and they want to spend as much time with him as they can. My father asks to spend an afternoon with me on Monday, and Peggy and I are planning to clean out a storage unit near our previous home in Florida at some point, but other than that, the trip will be about spending time together.

On Sunday evening, Joe and my parents retire for the evening at around 9 p.m. I ask Peggy what Mike said he observed about Joe. Peggy tells me Mike noticed the same things she did but that he also thought Joe wasn't as accurate in remembering historical sports events as he used to be and sometimes had the information somewhat confused. He said Joe understands what's going on around him despite the memory changes.

"Mike is so glad that he came to see Joe, and he wants to enjoy spending time together while Joe can communicate as well as he can," she adds. "He loves Joe, and they've become friends over the years. He's always looked forward to playing golf with Joe on the holidays and vacations we shared."

As Peggy talks, I remember the many times and places they've played golf together—North Carolina, South Carolina, Lake Placid, Naples, West Palm Beach, Jupiter, Daytona, and Lakeland, to name a few. The men in the family often played golf together in the summer and around Thanksgiving, and Christmas. Joe and Mike are good golfers, and they've always enjoyed a camaraderie yet a competitive spirit when they play.

◆

Our time in Florida flies by. On Monday afternoon, I show my father around the area, including the golf courses, the beach, and the small town we live in. I haven't explored much, so I welcome the opportunity to familiarize myself with the area and some time with my father. I'm comfortable with Joe staying with Peggy and my mother while we spend the afternoon together.

I drive to the nearest golf club and we sit on benches overlooking the driving range and talk. Until I heard him talking, I didn't realize that my father was trying to get me away from the house so he could speak to me alone and that he really wasn't all that interested in touring the area.

"Lynn, I know this will be hard for you to hear," he says. "I can't begin to imagine what you're going through, but I can imagine how I would feel if it were your mom with this illness."

He tells me that now that he's seeing Joe for the first time, he's noticed some differences—mostly physically but a little mentally—but that Joe is still himself. He notes that Joe still has his sense of humor and understands what's going on.

"I have a friend from our church who's a doctor; in fact, he's a neurosurgeon," he continues. "When you first told us about Joe, I started talking to him about the diagnosis. So, if you'll let me, I want to tell you what he told me. Okay?" he asks. I nod, and he continues talking.

"I told him about the type of glioma Joe has, the treatment he's undergoing, and the clinical trial," my dad tells me. "In his opinion, Joe has limited time—much more limited than you've told us—and that he'll be surprised if Joe makes it past Christmas this year."

Noticing my reaction of shock, he quickly adds, "Now, wait a minute, please. I'm telling you this so you can prepare for what's to come. The timeline may be off a little, but it's very unlikely that Joe has years in front of him."

I must say, I'm astounded. Christmas—this year? What?! No way. Joe has to be with me much longer than that. I can't be without him so soon—just six months from now. We're moving here so we can enjoy some retirement time together. We both want it and need it so much.

"Dad, I appreciate what you're telling me and that you know someone who has knowledge about this type of illness," I reply. "But your friend has never even seen Joe and doesn't know the specifics. And on the Internet, it says some people live three to five years.* So that's what we're planning for. Joe is recovering, although he does have some short-term memory issues to work on. Christmas, *this year*—not possible!"

My dad has this way of looking at you with his dark blue eyes that can get a steely look to them. I see that look now.

"Lynn, I don't want to be telling you this," he says. "Believe me, this is the last thing I want to be doing. But you need to prepare yourself. I know you have your hands full taking care of Joe and selling your house in Connecticut so you can move here. There are more things you need to know about. As Joe's illness continues, his mental capability and his ability to manage his motor functions will weaken. He'll begin to lose control of bodily function gradually, and he won't be able to feed himself or talk."

"What is this conversation we're having?" I think to myself. "The doctors at MGH haven't told me any of this. Why not? I'll ask at our next appointment there."

I say, "Dad, I know you haven't seen Joe since his surgery and you may see things that I overlook because I'm with him every day. But I don't think he'll be at that point anytime soon. You can see he's walking without help, although he's slower than he used to be. And yes, his balance is off a little, but it's nothing he can't manage. He isn't playing golf, because a full swing affects his balance, but otherwise he's pretty stable."

I tell him our plan is to move to Florida in September so we're not in the Northeast for another winter, assuming we sell our house in Connecticut. I'll explain that we'll be staying with Greg when we go to Boston for treatment twice a month and that this trip was a way to confirm whether that would be feasible.

"I appreciate what you're telling me, Dad," I tell him, "but I think we're okay now."

"I understand what I'm telling you is a shock," my dad says. "But my friend is pretty good at what he does. And he tells me that this isn't something anyone survives—no one, no matter what. Most people survive eight to fourteen months, and the degradation is fast once it starts.

"I know this is hard to hear, but you need to start making decisions," he continues. "Not to be too blunt, but have you and Joe decided where he'll rest? If not, you need to talk about it."

Well, of course we haven't discussed it yet. I pause as I remember Joe's latest MRI results. The doctor was hinting, no more than hinting, that Joe's treatment may need to change. He wants Joe to have another MRI in one month instead of two. I'm trying to take things as they come, not think about Joe being gone. He can't leave; I can't be without him. He's my only real love, the one person I trust with everything in my life, the one I can always count on to provide balance to the world—he can't leave. I just can't imagine a world where I don't wake up beside him every morning.

I respond, "Okay, Dad, I appreciate what you're saying. And I'll talk to Joe's doctors at his next appointment and see what I find out."

I explain that I've asked the doctors about disease progression but they haven't given me any details except to say they'll help me with that when the time comes. But no specifics.

"Thank you for talking to me about this, Dad," I tell him.

He nods and we stay seated on the bench at the golf course for a little while, watching the golfers practice. I think to myself, "Joe is going to be here on the range soon, I know it."

Joe, Peggy, and Mom are sitting in the TV area when we return. Dad and I did a little driving around before we came back to the house and we describe what we saw. Joe says he'd like to drive to the golf course and look around one of the days we're here, so we agree to do that.

◆

The next few days proceed with a family closeness surrounding us each day. We share the everyday tasks around the house, and we don't do much cooking as we either order food to pick up or go out to a restaurant. One afternoon, Peggy and I drive to a storage unit in Jupiter to clear out the contents, including items saved from Joe's parents' house. Before we leave, I consult with Joe about what to keep, and he says he doesn't want any of it. Okay, now we know what to do.

It's 90 degrees and sunny in South Florida. We get to the storage unit at around 10 a.m. There are no dumpsters in the storage area, so we need to find a place to dispose of items. But first we need to see what's in the storage unit. Fortunately, it's an air-conditioned unit, so it's reasonably comfortable when we sort through the items. Peggy and I start opening boxes and quickly see that there are many family memorabilia items that someone might want to keep, such as Joe's father's college diploma, pictures from his time in World War II, prints from Japan, and photographs of people we don't recognize but that another family member might. So we spend several hours going through everything and packing up family memorabilia to send to any of Joe's relatives who might want them. There's a double bed mattress and box springs that need to be discarded, boxes of old birthday and Christmas cards collected over the years, and boxes of newspaper cuttings with recipes, obituaries, and articles that have been saved. We pack the items into Peggy's SUV and make several trips to leave them at the municipal dump.

Peggy is such a help to me, and I couldn't have done this job by myself. Even with two of us managing the double bed mattress, a few less-than-gracious words escaped my mouth while we struggle to get it into the SUV. The dump is particularly revolting, and we don't waste (no pun intended) one second getting in and out of the area. But we manage, and the storage unit is finally cleared out.

Joe's favorite place in the house is the screened lanai. Every day, he takes a seat in one of the Cape Cod-style composite chairs with a view of the water, the birds, and the nearby building construction and revels in the warm humid summer breeze. Sometimes when I look out at him, I see him dozing a little. On our last morning, I open the door to see how he's doing. Joe gives me a lazy smile and asks me to join him, so I take a seat.

"What are we waiting for to move here?" he says. "Our sixteen-year business trip to Connecticut is over. I love it here and don't want to spend any more time in Connecticut. I think I can manage the travel back and forth for treatment. Sitting here every day looking out over the water is so relaxing. I feel like I'm where I belong again. Let's get down here as soon as we can."

It's music to my ears: I feel the same way.

◆

The Florida trip was a success. We feel we can manage the trip going back and forth to Boston for treatment. My family will be much closer to us in Florida, which will be helpful. I haven't forgotten what my father talked to me about, and at Joe's next infusion treatment at MGH, I ask questions about what to expect. I also scour the Internet for information.

Unfortunately, it turns out that Dad's friend wasn't far off. I learn from an online search that common end-of-life symptoms for people with brain cancer include severe fatigue and weakness, problems eating, problems with digestion and bodily functions, vomiting, difficulty swallowing, breathing problems, confusion, agitation, and depression.* At Joe's appointment before his immunotherapy treatment, after bloodwork and a review of the results, I follow Nurse N out of the room so I can talk to her without Joe present. I tell her that I'm worried about Joe's last MRI results and that I'd like to know what to look for that might indicate tumor progression. And of course, she tells me what we're always told.

"Well, anything that changes," she replies. "A seizure, balance issues, change in appetite, nausea—things like that."

I decide to take what I consider to be a more straightforward approach. "What I'm asking is, what will happen to Joe when the disease progresses?"

Once again, I get a vague "we'll cross that bridge when we come to it" type of response. I feel so stupid. Am I wording the question in an unclear way? Am I asking something inappropriate? Why can't I get a direct answer to a direct question?

I try again: "What are the steps that Joe will go through as this disease progresses?"

"It depends on where the disease spreads, but his motor control function and brain function will eventually become impaired," she answers. "We'll continue to monitor him through clinical evaluation and MRI tests."

Nurse N excuses herself, saying she needs to see another patient. I guess I got some kind of answer, but I don't really understand.

The house in Connecticut is on the market. The third bedroom is complete, thanks to Ray and Al. We've received the required permits, passed inspection, paid the taxes, and listed it with the real estate agent. There's interest in the house, and showings begin mid-June. Our wills and financial planning are also complete. We have a plan and we're sticking to it.

Our friends Cheryl and Jim have kept up with Joe and his progress throughout Joe's illness. They're parents to Andrew, who helped us so much by taking care of things at home while we were in Boston. Jim golfs frequently, and Joe used to play with him regularly. They visited Joe a couple of times before we left for Florida, and they come to see us again when we return to Connecticut.

Jim and Cheryl are also planning to relocate to Florida, and we discuss subjects like selling our houses, packing, and transporting cars to another state. We compare our experiences with real estate agents and talk about the best moving companies to use. We're trying to relocate a couple of months sooner than they are, but the process is the same. It's so helpful to discuss all the things that need to be accomplished, as moving is one of life's major and most stressful events. Joe's illness is the priority, and moving is secondary, so the move is being executed over a six-month period. Eventually, the packing, sorting, and clearing out of items is accomplished. I'm getting estimates from moving companies, including rates on household items and cars.

This leads to a discussion about automobiles. Right now, we have two —one for Joe and one for me. We haven't used Joe's car much in six months as he's not driving. I occasionally drive Joe's car to Boston or the grocery store, to be sure to utilize the car. But we don't really need both cars since Joe isn't driving. But it's a major defeat to actually take the step of downsizing to one car. It implies that Joe isn't going to drive a car again, although neither of us has given up. I'm not exactly sure how to approach this with Joe, but I decide a practical discussion including costs of maintaining two cars is the best way.

"Joe, the quotes I'm getting for moving the cars is close to $2,000 for both," I tell him. "Also, we're carrying car insurance and being taxed in Connecticut for both cars. We really aren't using both very much."

Joe is sitting in the sunroom on the sofa and I'm on the loveseat. When he turns to look at me, his expression changes from one of interest to one of sadness. Even his dark brown eyes sadden. It breaks my heart, and I wonder if I'm doing the right thing. He doesn't respond, so I try again.

"Joe, we have a car in Florida," I say. "I know it's older and that we should sell this car, but when we move, where will we park all three cars? Your car is leased, so why don't we return it and ship my car down to Florida? If you start driving again, you can drive mine and we can always buy a car once we're there if we need two cars."

I get up and sit next to him. I lean next to him and hold his right hand, resting my head on his shoulder.

Joe continues to be quiet for a few minutes until he shrugs and says, "I know it needs to be done. I'm not driving, and I shouldn't be. It's too risky—not just for me, but for other drivers as well. And I understand we're wasting money when our income has been reduced. But I'm not giving up—I just don't feel well enough to drive right now."

I nod in agreement.

Then his hand tightens on mine and he sighs, "I've been driving since I was sixteen. Feels like one more thing that I'm losing."

I stay with Joe in the sunroom. I don't want him to see the tears slowly running down my cheeks as he talks. Once again, he doesn't complain, but what a loss of independence it must be for him. Being sick and gradually losing what you had totally sucks. My thoughts, not his. I fight to diffuse the anger and resentment I feel rising in me.

I desperately want to blame something, someone, for his situation. But there's no one to blame, and that would be a misguided use of energy anyway.

Chapter 6: Setback

Though wise men at their end know dark is right,
Because their words had forked no lightning they
Do not go gentle into that good night.

Dylan Thomas

On the evening of June 27, I'm partially reclined on the sofa in the living room, watching TV. I hear Joe walking slowly from the bedroom, shuffling his feet very slightly. I sit up when I hear him approaching, and I look over my shoulder to see him holding his right side with his left hand as he slowly sits down in the grog chair.

"Lynn, my stomach hurts," he says. "It really hurts."

I walk over to him and ask, "Can you tell me *where* your stomach hurts?"

I immediately wonder if it's his appendix causing the pain, as I had mine removed in the fall of 2015. Joe says it hurts on his right side. Oh no, I think to myself. I ask him several questions and find out that it started when he lay down in bed, he doesn't feel like he has gas, and he feels a little bit better when he's lying down than when he's sitting or standing. I suggest that he go back to the bedroom to lie down, and I help him up from the chair. I don't know what to make of it, but I know he wouldn't be telling me about it if he weren't in serious pain—he has a high threshold for pain.

We walk side by side through the hallway to our bedroom. As we turn the corner, Joe starts to fall, his knees buckling. It happens so quickly that I instinctively slide under his upper body to soften his fall and try to keep him from hitting his head. His eyes are closed, and he appears to have lost consciousness. He didn't hit his head, thank God. I gently slide out from under him, rest his head down carefully, and place a pillow from the bed under his head. Then I grab the phone on the nightstand and call 911 for help.

I talk to Joe while he's lying on the floor, telling him that help is coming. I tell him over and over that it will be all right, that I love him, and that he's going to be taken care of. I finally hear the ambulance siren after what seems like an eternity, but it's actually been only ten minutes. Joe opens his eyes shortly before the ambulance arrives and continues to say how badly his stomach hurts. I run to the door and let the EMT in. They take Joe's vital signs before they put him on a stretcher. Then they navigate the front door, the rain-splattered steps, and the driveway and put him in the ambulance. They ask me whether I want to go to Manchester Memorial Hospital or St. Francis Hospital, and I tell them I'll follow them to St. Francis. I grab my windbreaker and purse, lock up the house, and catch up to the ambulance. I follow the ambulance as closely as I can, but I lose it when it veers off on an exit for EMT vehicles only to I-84W. I've never been to St. Francis Hospital, and I try to find it using my car navigation system. After a few tries, I have the address set and I drive through roads at night, relying only on the navigation system. I follow the signs to the emergency room, but I don't know where to park once there. I backtrack to find a place to park, run to the ER, and try to find Joe. I need to be sure the EMT understands Joe's medical history, although I tried to tell the ambulance team some of it as quickly as I could before they left.

I see an ambulance entrance and I run down the ramp to double doors, pushing them open and running in. An ambulance orderly sees me and tells me I can't use those doors. I say, "My husband was just brought in—please let me through! I need to explain his medical history!" I'm in a total crisis at this point, which I guess he can see, because he lets me in and directs me to an admittance area in the hospital. I ask where Joe is and they direct me to his ER staging room. I'm so anxious that I'm sure I seem to be out of control, yet when I enter Joe's room, I see that he's calm, quiet, and relaxed.

"Hey, Lynn, they gave me fentanyl!* I'm feeling *no* pain," he says. "Whew...they gave it to me in the ambulance, and it really helped." He's talking slowly and softly, with a lazy, slightly lopsided half-smile on his lips. I pull a chair to his bedside and hold his hand while he closes his eyes and rests.

Joe is reasonably comfortable in the private emergency room. The fentanyl continues to numb him. I sit in an uncomfortable upholstered chair on rollers without wheel locks. The room is brightly lit, the walls a dirty-beige color, the floor in need of cleaning. I'm impatient for a doctor to visit Joe. What's wrong? Why is he in such pain? We wait for close to two hours before an ER doctor enters the room. I describe what happened and explain Joe's medical history, and then the doctor asks Joe questions. He does a clinical diagnostic evaluation, pressing his hands on various places on Joe's abdomen, trying to determine the source of the pain and feel for obstructions and abnormalities. He determines the general area of pain but finds nothing else. He orders a CT scan of Joe's abdomen as the next step. He hasn't yet admitted Joe to the hospital, so we stay in the ER patient room.

It's now 4 a.m., and I continue to be uncomfortable sitting in the rollaway chair. But Joe continues to rest and is in a light sleep. I try to doze a little bit, but I can't really relax. This is so surreal. I'm worried that it's a side effect of Joe's immunotherapy treatment, though I don't recall seeing anything about it from the disclaimer Joe signed. I close my eyes and focus on positive things, like knowing Joe is being taken care of in the hospital where they'll find out what's happening.

◆

I'm in an empty burgundy carpeted room with several suitcases around me, stuffing clothes into the suitcases without even folding them. Clothes I don't recognize, with all kinds of bright prints colored in red and blue, are in my hand. The windows are closed and dark. Tears are running down my face. Joe—where's Joe? I need him to come back, to talk to me—why did he leave? I remember him leaving, and I don't think he's coming back. Why? I'm sobbing almost uncontrollably. I stand and start to leave the room. The door is open— an extraordinarily tall door, painted white, with raised panels. For some reason, I look behind to door. There he is! There's Joe! But his face is gaunt, his eyes so very dark, set in skin with a grayish taint. He's looking at me, staring so seriously at me. Then we're on a hilly golf course, the green below. As we approach the green, several golfers raise their hands to greet Joe. He responds, and like the other golfers, we lie down on our bellies in the high grass around the green and watch the players on the green. Joe reaches for my hand and clasps it tightly. Our eyes meet and we smile at each other. Joe looks suntanned in the afternoon light; his hair is salt-and-pepper gray, and his eyes are warm. We're having fun spying on the golfers below. The last golfer makes a chip shot, but it doesn't reach the green because it hits a sand trap rake. Joe says, "What a rakish shot!"

I'm startled from my dream state by a hospital orderly who's coming to take Joe for his CT scan. I feel disoriented as I look around and quickly remember where I am and what's happening. Joe wakes from his light sleep and waves his right hand to the orderly, calling him "Captain."

"Captain, where are we off to this morning?" he says.

It's now close to 7 a.m. The orderly explains where he's taking Joe and tells me he'll be back in an hour or so. He advises me to wait in the room, so I use the time to contact Greg and Joe's brother and sister. I explain the situation and tell them I'll be back in touch when I know more.

I'm so anxious and uneasy about Joe as I continue to wonder, "Is this related to the clinical trial drug?" I hope the CT scan will give us some answers. I walk to the hospital cafeteria to get something to eat while Joe is gone. I decide to eat there because I don't know if the smell of food will bother him if he has returned from his CT scan. I sit in a brown plastic chair with shiny metal legs and back support. The table is a speckled tan pattern and needs to be wiped off before I eat. It's a small cafeteria, but the breakfast selection is decent enough. It's not too crowded, but there are enough people around to make it a little bit noisy. As I eat, I remember the tricks Joe would play on me in the kitchen while I prepared breakfast before work.

> I'm always rushing in the morning before I leave for work, and today is no different. My routine is to go to the gym at 5 a.m., swim laps , return home, dress for work, and eat quickly. If I stay on task, I can be at work no later than 8 a.m. I'm in the kitchen and just put my oatmeal in the microwave to cook. I turn to the countertop adjacent to the sink and start slicing peaches, an apple, and a banana to add to my oatmeal. Joe walks in to the kitchen and takes a diet soda from the refrigerator. Breakfast of champions…I hear the pantry door and a kitchen cabinet open behind me as I turn around to get

> my oatmeal out of the microwave. But the microwave is empty. Where's my oatmeal? I'm in a rush and figure that maybe I forgot to make it. Joe is now sitting at the dining table opening the newspaper and starting to eat breakfast of his own. I stare at him for a minute. Did he do it to me *again?* All right, I'll play along. Where's my oatmeal? I look in the pantry: not there. I open each cabinet: not there. Okay, maybe I didn't really cook it. I walk around behind Joe, just checking around him. Can't find it….
>
> I finally concede and ask, "Joe, did you see the oatmeal I was cooking?" I hate doing that, because I can't be sure if he moved it.
>
> He looks at me so innocently and says, "Oh, were you making oatmeal this morning?"
>
> Now I know for sure that he's moved it. I decide to look at the chair seats near him, and what do you know—there it is, a bowl of oatmeal!
>
> "Ha!" I exclaim. "I can't believe you did it to me again! And I fell for it!"
>
> Joe laughs and says, "It was easy today—you were so busy with the fruit chopping that you didn't even see me move the bowl. Gotcha! Gotta run though. Have a good fun day today!"
>
> He winks as he gets up to leave. This is not a daily sabotage, but something that has been a recurring event over the years. I never know when he'll try to pull it on me again.

I finish eating and return to Joe's room at about the same time he's brought back from his CT scan. We're told that the doctor will stop by later and let us know the results. Joe isn't in as much pain as he was earlier, but he looks apprehensive when he comes in to the room. Neither of us knows what to think at this point. We wait several hours before a team of gastrointestinal doctors finally step into the room. They check his vital signs, complete a clinical evaluation, and ask him about his pain level. They explain that although the CT scan isn't showing any problems, it can't necessarily find all potential problems. They confirm that it's not his appendix. They want him to try to drink something and will decide the next steps depending on the results. They give him some liquid, but he can't keep anything down. They then decide to admit him for observation.

Joe's single-patient room in St. Francis Hospital is very nice, with large windows, an engineered hardwood floor, and a private bathroom. But there are no accommodations for me to spend the night—at least not on any kind of bed. The hospital wing doctor stops by to see Joe at around 6 p.m. There's no change in his condition, and he still can't keep anything down. To keep him hydrated, they set up an IV in his left hand. Joe and I continue to be very worried, but what can we do at this point? The gastrointestinal team will visit him in the morning, with rounds beginning at 6 am.

The gastro team stops by Joe's room at around 7:30 a.m. I'm waiting to see them, full of questions. I don't understand the rationale behind this "observation" thought process. Joe isn't eating or drinking, and I'm worried about his strength, although he's in much less pain. Once again, a clinical test is performed but reveals nothing new. Joe still can't hold any liquids down, so the doctors decide to have a G-tube inserted in his stomach to remove any digestive fluids that might be accumulating.* They're very nervous about his medical history and are hesitant to do any type of exploratory surgery, not knowing how he'll react to anesthesia and the healing process from surgery. No one knows what's wrong; nobody can tell us why this is happening. They ask for contact information for Joe's doctors at MGH so they can discuss options for Joe's treatment, and I gladly provide it.

It goes on and on. It's now been four days in the hospital with Joe under observation. There's been no change at all, and he hasn't eaten since the night he was admitted. The doctors at St. Francis explain that gastrointestinal issues will often resolve themselves—there can be a "lazy bowel" that will self-correct over time. Because of Joe's glioma, exploratory surgery could be very risky. I ask about Joe's diet, concerned that he's only receiving liquids; it doesn't seem like enough nutrition to me. They confer for several hours until they finally agree to have him fed intravenously through a PICC line, so they send a team to Joe's room to insert it.* He still has a G-tube inserted in his stomach. The G-tube continuously removes bile, which indicates that he has some sort of blockage or obstruction that wasn't visible on the CT scan.

I ask the doctors about the results of the conversation with Joe's team at MGH, but they tell me they haven't been able to find a time when all the doctors are available for a discussion. So we've been waiting four days and the doctors haven't found a way to connect with each other yet? I call Dr. D at MGH and explain the situation. I also try to reach the gastro team at St. Francis to arrange a discussion. In addition, I send records to each hospital so they can share information, yet it still takes two more days for the doctors to confer. The two facilities use the same electronic system to share patient data and can send information to each other directly, but it's actually more efficient if I get a copy of Joe's patient records from St. Francis and have them delivered overnight to MGH.

Once MGH sends Joe's records to St. Francis electronically, the doctors confer. They conclude that Joe is a high risk for surgery. They say the issues he's having now seem unrelated to his immunotherapy treatment, but they can't be certain until the obstruction clears. So, Joe continues under observation with the hope that the condition will remedy itself. Sometimes intestines that have become twisted can somehow untwist themselves and relieve an obstruction, and the gastro team is hoping that'll happen for Joe.

It's hard for me to believe that once or twice a day, I'm reduced to a blubbering, teary-eyed, snot-congested, drama queen of a wife. Desperate to stop the unstoppable, persistently demanding optimal comfort, all the while trying to process the contrast between what was and what is. The walls start to close in and a growing, escalating, all-consuming panic seeps through. I search for a way to head off the loss of perspective and alleviate the emotional pain. I quickly leave the room while Joe sleeps, curled to one side, his whimpers almost silent. All I can think about is making it all stop—getting our lives back and moving forward together. But it will never be, I think pessimistically.

I walk toward the parking garage, though I have no intention of leaving. I ask at the information desk if there's a park or garden nearby. There isn't. I walk through the public garage, circle to the left, and take a seat on the only unoccupied bench in a small outside seating area. I take deep breaths and try to control the flow of tears. An abdominal obstruction on top of stage 4, unmethylated, astrocytoma glioma is quickly accelerating Joe's already deteriorating condition. He's so brave and uncomplaining as this horrible disease continues to worsen. It breaks my heart to be completely unable to stop the progression. It gives new meaning to the phrase "feeling useless."

I'm abusing my family with the persistent phone calls, searching for the pain to stop, if only for a few minutes. Just craving a way to offload feelings of what is to come, and what I see every day. We know the life expectancy is about six to fourteen months. We know there's no cure—not even an FDA-approved effective treatment. My husband, so full of life, subtle, complex humor, not himself yet only wanting to please. My husband, my very best friend in the world, my confidante, my touchstone, short on life.

In the process of sending records to MGH from St. Francis, I become acquainted with "W," the lead hospital document control manager. I explain our circumstances and Joe's primary health issue, the glioma. I see her face stiffen and darken as I continue describing his story. When I finish, W is immediately helpful and focused on communication with MGH. After the doctors confer on Joe's situation, I return to her station to thank her. She tells her colleagues that she's taking a short break and asks me to step into the hallway. "Uh-oh, I guess I was too pushy and she's going to let me have it," I think to myself. When she turns to me, I see her eyes slightly misting.

Instead, W tells me her father had a glioma and passed away about a year ago. She takes a deep breath and tells me the disease is an ugly, ugly illness and the progression is truly horrific. She helped with her father's care and knows firsthand the unspeakable advancement and the loss of capability that comes with it. W says he received excellent care at Yale New Haven Hospital, and she offers to give me contact information for a support group for glioma patients. I've felt so alone in caring for Joe, other than the terrific help I've gotten from MGH. This is the first offer of organized emotional support that I've gotten, connecting me with others in similar circumstances. She gives me a phone number and name to contact for more information and for volunteers to talk to me at any time if it will help. I can see that it's difficult for her to discuss and that she's opening up a wound that was starting to heal by talking to me. It's so very kind of her to offer to help me at her own expense, and I thank her for her help.

The days are long, and Joe's pain from the G-tube is continuously increasing. It's hard for him to talk with the tube in place, and his throat is dry and sore. I visit the hospital chapel every day, constantly praying for his self-recovery. For the first time since his glioma diagnosis, I start to realize I'm losing him. Really, it's happening. And I'm completely powerless to help him. Yes, I can be his advocate. Yes, I can be with him, love him every second of the day. Yes, I can beg God to spare him, to heal him, to give us more time together. I do believe in the power of prayer. But I also know that what I want is not necessarily aligned with the overall plan for Joe and me. And I don't get to decide the plan. I have to accept it. Well, f*** that. I don't know how to accept it, but I sure know how to fight it. And fight I will.

After observing Joe for eighteen days, the gastro team decides that the intestinal blockage is unlikely to resolve on its own and that surgery should be performed. It will be both exploratory and corrective, if possible, and will be completed laparoscopically.* At this point, Joe has missed one of his scheduled immunotherapy infusion treatments, and we don't yet know whether he'll be allowed to continue with it. The risks of surgery versus the risks of continuing the "wait and see" perspective without the blockage correcting itself suggests that surgery is the best path at this point. The MGH doctors concur, so surgery it is. It'll start with exploratory laparoscopy of the right side of Joe's stomach area. Depending on what is found, the problem may be corrected by lifting out a small section of the intestine and straightening it out. If it's a large obstruction, the intestines could possibly require a resection, which could mean a longer incision to repair. The surgery could be anywhere from two to five hours.

◆

It's Sunday, July 17—the night before Joe's surgery. I sit next to him, continuing to read the same book aloud that I've been reading to him the entire time he's been in St. Francis, at his request. The book, "Shakespeare" by Bill Bryson, is one that Greg gave him for Christmas. It has helped Joe take his mind off the pain from the G tube and has helped him through the last few weeks. I don't know how much he actually listened to, as he often closed his eyes soon after I started to read. The TV is turned on and set to a music channel playing soft, soothing piano music in the background.

Once again, I ask a chaplain to come to Joe's room to administer the sacrament of anointing of the sick to provide courage, comfort, and strength for the upcoming surgery. Joe can barely talk, but he thanks the chaplain for coming to see him. He's so much weaker than he was when he was admitted to the hospital, and I'm terrified that I'll lose him during the surgery. I give him a kiss before the orderly moves his bed from the patient room to the operating wing of the hospital. I can't go with him to the operating room, but I have directions to a small waiting area near the surgical room. I'm resigned to the outcome, preparing myself for the worst. How can Joe muster the stamina for so much physical trauma in a seven-month period?

The waiting area isn't crowded, and it's hard for me to sit quietly. I walk around the waiting area, pace the corridors, and eventually settle on a padded bench outside. I have my great-grandmother's rosary beads with me, now looking worn out through many years of use. This rosary is my constant companion since Joe's initial diagnosis in January. I touch the beads and pray over and over for Joe to have the strength to survive and recover from this surgery. I don't know whether my prayers will be answered, but I do believe that what is best for Joe will happen.

I don't know how much time has passed. In the periphery of my right eye, I see a pristine white floating material and realize a doctor is quietly approaching along the carpeted hallway. I look up and make eye contact with him and we recognize each other: it's Dr. G. He sits to the left of me on the bench and says softly, "It was what I suspected: the intestine was twisted and causing an obstruction."

Dr. G explains that he made a small incision and pulled the intestine out, straightened it, and set it back in place. He says he didn't need to resect any tissue, so the procedure was as minor as possible.

"Your husband is doing well and is in the recovery room," he tells me. "We'll keep him there overnight, so I suggest you go home and come back in the morning to see him.

I tell the doctor I don't want to leave Joe, so he tells me they'll call me in an hour or so to see him.

When I ask Dr. G if he knows how it may have happened, he shrugs and says there are many possible causes, such as a sharp movement or the digestive process—the exact cause is unknown. I ask if he thinks it may be related to Joe's immunotherapy treatment, but he says he's seen the same problem many times over the years in people who haven't undergone that type of treatment. He pauses before telling me he recently lost a close family member and understands how I must be feeling. He explains again that they were trying to avoid subjecting Joe to recovering from surgery because of his glioma, but that once he saw the cause of the blockage, he realized the problem wouldn't have self-corrected.

Dr. G then suggests that after I see Joe, I go home and try to rest. He assures me that Joe will be carefully watched and that I'll get a call if anything changes. I thank Dr. G for all he's done for us. The team tried so hard to avoid surgery to minimize Joe's risk and pain, but it proved necessary.

I call Greg and then Joe's brother and sister to let them know that Joe is in the recovery room and the surgery was successful. I also tell Jean, one of Joe's friends from work, so she can let his other friends know. She and two of Joe's other work friends, Jeanne and Mike, visited Joe twice in the hospital, which helped him tremendously. Although Joe was in a weakened state, their visits meant so much to him. They joked about work, told stories about people they all knew, and described the work hours and pressures. Each told Joe how much they missed him at work and how it wasn't the same without him. When they left, Joe told me how much he appreciated seeing them and how much it helped him.

I'm allowed to see Joe about an hour later. The first thing I notice is that the G-tube has been removed. The tube was Joe's nemesis for days on end, and I know that when he wakes up, he'll feel so much better without it. He's lying on his back, the intravenous feed tube and fluids line from surgery still in place, one in each arm. His color looks okay to me, and I ask his nurse how he's doing. She says he'll be coming out of the anesthetic soon and I can stay until he does. She also says his blood pressure and oxygen percentage* are stable and as expected.

I sit in a chair to Joe's right side and hold his hand, feeling the soft, dry palm, careful to not move his arm or the IV in it. I feel gratitude and thankfulness that he's with me still. Joe moves his head slightly, and I look at his face as his eyes open halfway. A half, somewhat lopsided smile forms on his lips. I immediately say, "Welcome back, Joe! Everything went well. They found the problem and corrected it. You're doing great!" The nurse, seeing that Joe is waking up, approaches his bed and asks if he'd like to have some water. He nods yes, so she holds the straw in the water cup to his lips and he takes a sip. He rests his head back on the pillow. "No, tube," he croaks. "I can swallow again." And that's all he can manage. I tell him that he'll stay in the ICU overnight and I'll see him first thing in the morning. I'm not sure if he hears me, because I think he's fast asleep already.

Over the next couple of days, Joe has some light food and keeps it down, and he's able to have a bowel movement. A hospital physical therapist comes by Tuesday afternoon and Wednesday morning and has Joe walking very slowly with a walker. It's decided that he'll need an RN and physical and occupational therapy when he goes back home, so the hospital coordinates with his primary care physician to have the claim submitted.

Joe is released from the hospital late Wednesday afternoon. I'm very surprised that he's ready to go so soon, but hospitals seem to release patients more quickly these days. I'm not totally comfortable with him leaving so soon, but it's not up to me. I understand the risk of infection in a hospital, and I respect the doctor's decision to release Joe. I'm amazed at how quickly his strength is returning—he can already stand somewhat upright and shuffle around a bit. He seems to be balanced but does need someone with him when he walks around. I'm given instructions for caring for his incision, helping him shower, and watching out for signs of infection. Joe isn't on a restricted diet, but it's recommended that he gradually return to his regular diet. The hospital staff helps Joe get into the car from the wheelchair that is used to transport him from his room to the car, and we're on our way home.

◆

It's Sunday, July 25, and Joe has been home for four days. He continues to recover from his surgery and has developed no unusual issues. An RN evaluated him on Thursday and recommended at-home occupational, speech, and physical therapy. The occupational and speech therapists have already visited, physical therapy will start on Monday. The process is much like what followed Joe's brain surgery in January, but it's a different team of specialists and we know a little more than we did the first time, making it easier all around. Joe's incision is healing on schedule, and he's had no fever or infection. He's eating well and moving around as expected.

Now our issue is that Joe missed two immunotherapy treatments. When I contact MGH, Dr. D's assistant tells me Joe is no longer part of the clinical trial because of that.

I also schedule a call with Dr. D.

"Hello, Lynn. How are you? And how is Joe?" he asks.

I update Dr. D about Joe's status and tell him he should be able to travel in a couple of weeks.

After a long pause, Dr. D says, "It's so unfortunate that this happened to Joe. The clinical trial protocol is very strict, and it hasn't been followed as required. I understand that the intestinal blockage wasn't related to the clinical trial or his cancer, but at this point, he's no longer part of the trial. I can recommend that he continue in the trial, but the decision is no longer mine. I'll do what I can."

"So, Dr. D, what are Joe's treatment next steps then?" I ask quietly.

He suggests that I contact his office when Joe can travel and we can then discuss the options that we had talked about in June. He says he'll petition the clinical trial board but that we shouldn't count on the outcome being positive. He's very kind, and I understand what he's saying, but I'm terribly upset. I thank him for his help and time before we hang up.

Joe is very upset about the news also. We feel sure that the clinical trial would be Joe's best chance for remission,* as his particular type of glioma is so aggressive. It's bad enough that the intestinal blockage was such a painful ordeal for Joe, but on top of that, it affected his participation in the clinical study. I relay to Joe the conversation I had with Dr. D.

"The door isn't completely closed yet, at least," Joe says. "I know it's not likely that the decision will be reversed, but Dr. D says he's going to discuss it with the protocol board. I can only believe that something will come of it."

Joe is so objective and logical. He chooses to be an optimist and change course only when he has to. He has resolved that he won't worry yet and will wait for a final answer. I'm not of the same mindset, but I'm so thankful to have his guiding perspective.

It's said that bad things happen in groups of three. I know it's not based on fact—it's just a superstition, and I can't explain how it originated. But I do know that on top of the intestinal blockage and the potential disqualification from the clinical trial, a third problem surfaced for us: our real estate agent tells us that the potential buyer had rescinded the offer on our house. We'd gotten a reasonable offer while Joe was in the hospital, and we accepted. It was a bright moment in an otherwise bleak time. So I can't begin to express how the news spiraled me almost into a state of despair. What else can go wrong? Our plan was to leave for Florida in September so we didn't have to spend another cold winter in Connecticut. But it may not happen after all, as it seems we'll have to continue showing the house and try to get another offer.

Greg visits for the weekend, which is always an upbeat experience for all of us. He frequently traveled to visit Joe in the hospital, and he's pleased to see his father doing so much better at home without that horrible G-tube. The tube was necessary, but it was so painful, and thankfully it's gone now.

Colin stops over, and the three of us continue cleaning out the basement, taking turns staying with Joe. I make it sound like babysitting, but it's anything but: in reality, we all want to spend time with him. The basement is almost completely organized, but our timeline may be different now that we don't have a buyer for our house. But then I start to wonder if that's true. We can still leave in September as we planned even if the house isn't sold, can't we? It wouldn't be ideal for us—after all, we don't want to manage two homes, especially not one from a distance. But I start considering sticking with our original plan. It makes me feel better, at least. And so many things are already in motion. I have a moving van lined up. And a portable moving and storage container. And car transportation. And one-way tickets for us. Maybe we'll stay the course after all.

Joe's new physical therapist, "T," arrives at 10 a.m. on Monday. I lead T to the sunroom to meet Joe. He sits next to Joe and tells us about his background. He's married with two young children, is 6'5" and very fit, and enjoys triathlon training and marathon running—a manly man, so it appears. I can see that Joe immediately connects with him. T assesses Joe's strength and stamina and then defines a tailored physical plan to help him improve. He takes Joe outside for a walk to see how he does, first using his walker and then taking a few steps without. It's clear that Joe is really engaged and is enjoying the interaction with T.

For Joe, his physical improvement has largely depended on how he connects with people. He had this connection at MGH, and it looks like he's developing it with T now. He never found it at the facility in Connecticut, for whatever reason. After the assessment, T determines that he should meet with Joe twice a week, and he prepares daily "homework" for Joe to complete. The plan includes many exercises similar to those prescribed at MGH, plus walking every day. Physical therapy is off to a good start!

Well, I guess good things can happen in groups of three, also. Joe is so much stronger working under T's guidance. Once again, he's ready to practice his exercises and walk without me practically begging him to. And the results are apparent. He's walking again without his walker, although not as far as he was before his surgery. He's gradually becoming stronger, even though his left side still isn't as strong as his right. And he really enjoys talking to T about sports and current events while they walk and work out. I watch from the front steps as T guides him around the neighborhood. They're engaged in a conversation, and Joe is laughing. It's such a cliché, I know, but laughter really is the best therapy there is.

Our real estate agent continues to show our house to potential buyers. It's inconvenient, as we have to leave the house when it's being shown. We accommodate that by taking our walks in the park instead of around the neighborhood. After another four or five showings, we receive a second offer. I can't accept it fast enough. The closing date is at the end of September—not perfect, but very manageable. I'm so glad we didn't change our moving plans. We're headed for a departure mid-September!

My cell phone rings on Thursday afternoon. I don't recognize the number, but I recognize a Boston area code—it's Dr. D.

"I have some good news," he begins. "The clinical trial board has reevaluated Joe's condition and concur that his intestinal issue wasn't because of the clinical trial. They agree to have Joe reenter the program! Would Joe be able to be here on Wednesday?"

I'm astounded but immediately jubilant.

"Yes, of course we'll be there!" I exclaim. "Thank you so much. This means so much to us. I can't wait to tell Joe!"

After we hang up, I'm left staring at the phone in my hand. It's the best news ever! As I walk into the sunroom, Joe looks up from his tablet.

"What's up?" he asks, noticing the look on my face.

I lean over and hug him, and I tell him the news. We hold each other close and start crying. I never believed it would happen. But Joe did, and he was right to be optimistic. It's hard to explain the wave of relief being able to feel confident that once again, Joe will be receiving the best treatment available to him.

Joe and I sit together for the remainder of the afternoon, talking about the events of the last month. I feel emotionally battered having not expected Joe's intestinal blockage. For the first time, Joe describes his feelings.

"It feels like we've been on a roller coaster lately," he says. "We were on a path to move to Florida and had a good trial trip. Then there was my stint in St. Francis. Thank God that's over.

"I wish I knew what caused the blockage," he continues. "I guess we'll never know for sure. But it really was a big setback."

He acknowledges that he feels so much better and is getting stronger every day now that he's home. He says he wants to move as soon as possible and doesn't want to spend another winter in Connecticut.

He looks me in the eye and adds, "We haven't talked about a few things though that we need to. Lynn, I know neither of us wants to face the inevitable. Being in St. Francis and feeling as bad as I did really made me think about the short amount of time I may have. I'm not giving up, but….

"I don't have a bucket list or anything like that," he continues. "I'm with you and Greg, and that's what's most important to me. I'm also seeing my family, friends, and colleagues—some more than I have in a long time."

He pauses, and I hesitate before I ask, "Joe, where do you want to be after this is over? Do you want to be in Tennessee with your parents?"

He looks at me and says, "I want to be where you will be. As far as I'm concerned, funerals and burials are for the living. I don't really care where I'll be or what happens. I don't care about the service. Do what you think should be done. After all, I won't be here when it happens, right? As long as I'm with you."

"Joe, my parents have land in Lakeland and have offered us a place there if we want it," I tell him. "I know you just said you don't care, but would that be okay with you? I don't want to do anything you don't agree with."

He nods his head in agreement, and then I ask him, "Joe, is there anyone you want to see that you aren't in touch with, or anything in particular that you want to say to anyone that I can arrange for you to do?"

"No, other than some things I want to tell my brother," he replies. "I want him to know how much he means to me. I need to find the time to tell him sometime when he visits." I nod my head and continue to hold his hand tightly. I'm so happy that Joe's treatment at MGH is going to continue, but this conversation—especially initiated by Joe—is sobering. I study his face from the side view I have, but he's looking straight ahead and I can't read his expression. He looks tired to me—how could he not be after all he's been through? It's time for a little comic relief, and here comes our cat Rascal as if on cue. He enters the sunroom, eyeing Joe, with a meow-meow-meow. He jumps on Joe's lap and starts his loud purring and settling in. Joe pets him, and Rascal "smiles" back at him with his eyes while staring up at him. He starts kneading Joe's arm with his paws, his purring growing increasingly louder. Such a comforting kitty, always seeming to know when to reach out.

Our family, friends, and colleagues now know the timeline of our move. There are so many people who want to see Joe before we move, and it's a busy task arranging all the visits. Jean contacts me and suggests that a party be held in Joe's honor before we move. She tells me there are many people who want to see him and have missed him so much at work. It's a good idea, but I know Joe's stamina is limited. Jean and I discuss the options, and we decide that a lunch at Joe's regular golf course would be the best. We decide on a date, and Jean agrees to plan a seated, catered lunch in a private room where Joe will be able to remain sitting most of the time.

Joe has an MRI, a blood screening, and an appointment with Dr. D on August 2. His immunotherapy treatment resumes the following Wednesday, August 9. He missed a total of three immunotherapy treatments due to his intestine surgery and recovery. We follow our usual routine, traveling to Boston the night before the treatment and staying with Greg. We spend the next day at MGH, getting bloodwork and meeting with the clinical trial nurse and Dr. D. Nurse N isn't working today, so we see a new nurse. We miss seeing Nurse N as she's been with us throughout Joe's treatment, although we also work well with the new nurse. When Dr. D meets with Joe, he's especially thoughtful of Joe asking him about his recovery from surgery. He's a very caring physician, and Joe is touched by his interest. The bloodwork is within range to continue the treatment as planned, so we move to the 8th floor for Joe's infusion. We also have a different nurse for the infusion, as our usual nurse is on vacation. We miss her, too, but receive excellent care in her absence. The infusion process is finished in time for us to miss the workday traffic as we leave Boston, and we're back home in Connecticut by 5:30 p.m. It's a very long day for Joe, but as usual, he's not complaining. I can see that he's very tired, even though he doesn't say he is.

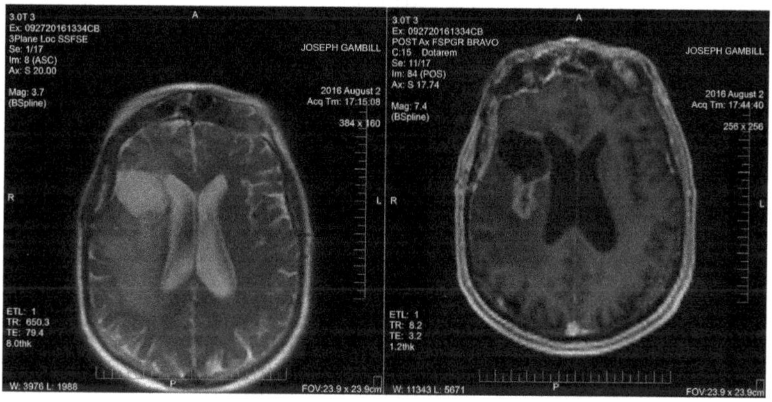

Our friends Jim and Cheryl visit us several times over the next few weeks before Joe and I move. They'll be relocating about a month after we plan to leave. We compare moving costs and plans and share ideas to make the moving process easier. It's a pleasant yet stressful time, knowing that we're so close to our goal of relocating. Joe is very excited to move, although he's sad to be leaving his work colleagues. He'll miss his work friends in Connecticut—both those who'll continue to work and those who've retired in the state. It's a bittersweet time, as an unexpected illness can turn your plans inside-out. Joe hadn't planned on retiring for several years.

◆

On Saturday, September 3, I turn right into the Topstone golf course parking lot, arriving early to find a parking spot as close to the clubhouse entryway as I can. Driving in, we see Jean parked in front of the clubhouse, unloading some boxes from her car. We wave as we drive past her and park the car. I get out of the car and walk around to the passenger side to help Joe get out. He's looking straight ahead, showing no signs of trying to stand up, so I ask him if he's okay.

Joe turns to me and says, "I hope no one asks me to stand up and give a speech. Sometimes at things like this, that happens. Please tell Jean I don't want to give a speech. I don't know what I'll say after all that's happened. I want people to remember me as dignified, not as foolish and sickly."

I assure him he won't be expected to give a speech, and I reach my hand out to help him stand up. But he waves me away, swinging his legs to the right and slowly standing up by himself. He's wearing khaki pants, a golf shirt, and a pullover windbreaker. We walk up the inclined walkway to the front steps of the clubhouse, where several golfers wave to Joe from the putting green.

"Hey, Joe!" one of them says. "Haven't seen you this summer—good to see you here. Hope we can play soon."

"Call me so we can play when you want," another says. "I'm looking forward to beating your sorry ass!"

Joe laughs, waves back, and retorts, "That'll be a first—you're on!"

On the way to the private room, we walk past the pro shop. The golf pro looks up as we're going by and waves at Joe. "Joe, where have you been all summer?" he says. "Hope you'll be playing here soon."

Joe waves back and says, "I plan on it. How are you hitting it?"

They exchange a few more pleasantries and we make our way to the private luncheon room. We walk past commemorative plaques from winners of past golf tournaments, and I see Joe's name on one of them.

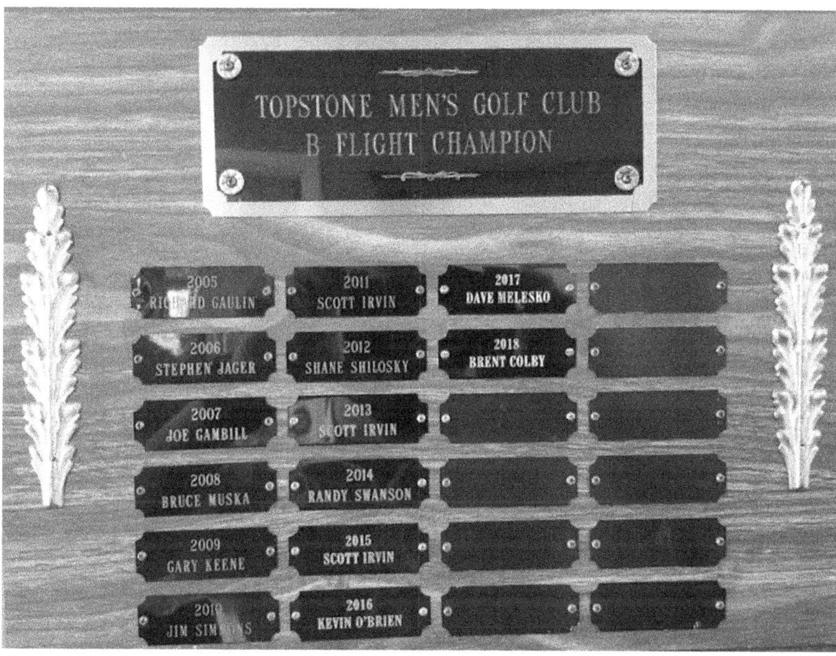

TOPSTONE MEN'S GOLF CLUB
B FLIGHT CHAMPION
2005
GAULIN
2006
STEPHEN JAGER
2007
JOE GAMBILL
2008
BRUCE MUSKA
2009
GARY KEENE
2011
SCOTT IRVIN
2012
SHANE SHILOSKY
2013
IRVIN
2014
RANDY SWANSON
2015
SCOTT IRVIN
2016
KEVIN O'BRIEN
2017
DAVE MELESKO
2018
BRENT COLBY

The room is set up with several round tables that seat six, covered by white tablecloths. In honor of the University of Tennessee, there are orange balloons tied to the centerpieces. At the front of the room is a long rectangular table covered with wrapped gifts and decorated with balloons. The room has a view of the eighteenth and tenth holes through the floor-to-ceiling windows. Golfers can be seen enjoying the well-manicured fairways and greens on this clear, sunny, 75-degree day. Jean and Jeanne walk over to Joe as he enters the room, and each gives him a hug. Jean looks closely at Joe's face and says she's so glad to see him. Both ask how he's feeling and tell him he looks great.

Mike, Joe's friend and office colleague, walks over to us and shakes Joe's hand.

"Good to see you, Joe. You're looking much better than the last time I saw you," he says, referring to the time he visited Joe at St. Francis.

Mike looks closely at Joe while he talks to him, measuring the change since he saw him last. Joe smiles, clearly in his element. He loves social occasions and being with people.

"Let's have a seat while the others arrive," Mike says.

There were so many people that wanted to attend, and Jean and I strategized on what to do. We ended up with 50 attendees, all current colleagues of Joe's from the department he's the technical fellow for. People from Puerto Rico, Florida, and Connecticut are attending. It's an informal affair, and there's a sense of excitement in the air.

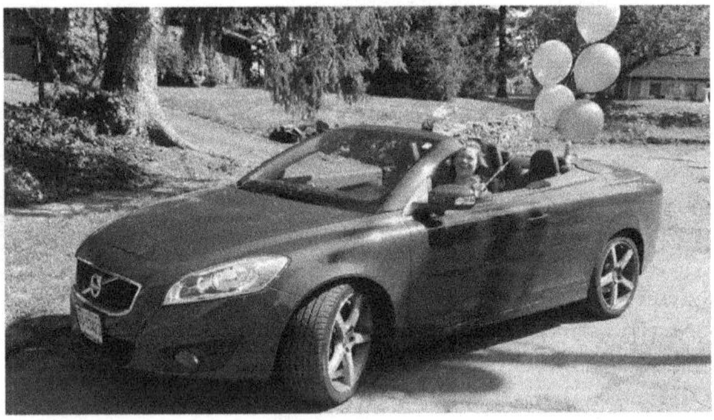

Knowing the nature of Joe's illness, we were careful to be sure that no "gawkers" would attend, trying to protect Joe as best we can.

As people enter the room, they approach Joe with smiling faces and wish him well, telling him how much they miss him at work, golf, or other events where they used to see him. They each express how good it is to see him and how sorry they are that he's moving. It's very touching to see. So many people care about Joe and truly value knowing him and working with him. The camaraderie in the room is palpable. Joe has worked on most of the company's military and commercial engines throughout the years and is a technical fellow with expertise in systems architecture. He designed and managed the design of most of the external hardware on our brand of engines flying today. He has two patents and countless successful designs in service and is known for his intellectual prowess both within the company and in our industry. He mentored many engineers over the years and is particularly proud that he's been able to give back through transfer of knowledge to so many. He was always eager to share his knowledge, understanding that the more information shared, the better the solution. Even with his intellect, he's quite humble and self-effacing. He never brags or boasts about his successes; instead, he lets the flying outcome speak for itself. It's one of the many reasons he's so well liked—that and his quick sense of observational humor.

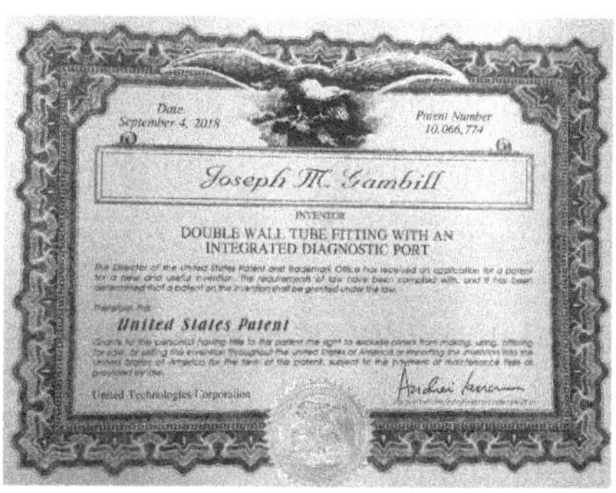
Date
September 4, 2018
Patent Number
10,066,774
Joseph M. Gambill
INVENTOR
DOUBLE WALL TUBE FITTING WITH AN
INTEGRATED DIAGNOSTIC PORT
United States Patent
United Technologies Corporation

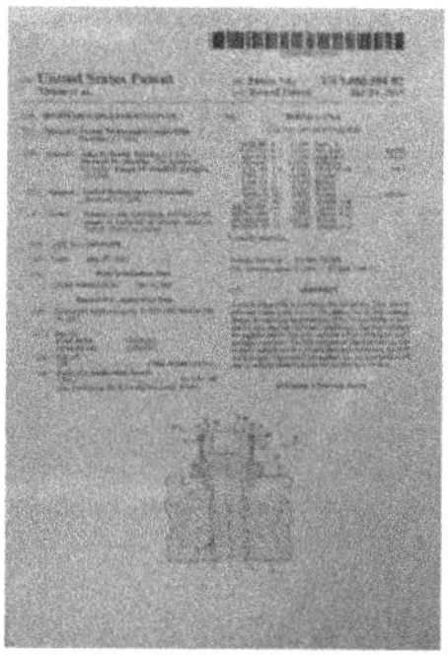

The luncheon is a large departure from Joe's current daily life. One of the side effects of Joe's condition is his ability to process some things. Conversations and interactions with people aren't a problem although they can be tiring for him, but things like time and schedules, continue to require more effort than they did before his illness. Being in familiar places is the best situation for Joe, which is why we have the luncheon at the golf club he's accustomed to. Once everyone arrives, the lunch buffet line is opened. Jean brings Joe a plate of food, while the guests serve themselves. Joe is surrounded by his closest colleagues at a front table, and they talk to Joe about the changes in the workplace while he's been gone. There've been many changes to staff, situations, locations, and management over the last nine months. Yes, nine months since Joe was at work, and so many people are here to be with him. After lunch, more fun unfolds.

Chris, who is Joe's supervisor, colleague, and friend, walks to the front of the room. He welcomes everyone and talks about today being a very special event to honor Joe as well as a send-off for him. He describes how working with Joe was such a pleasant experience, and he reminisces about meeting with Joe and how Joe supported his vision. He says Joe would say to him, "Chris, my job is to make your job easier." Chris also talks about Joe's value to the organization and his many accomplishments, including 37 years of service and being a systems architecture fellow, a manager for more than 25 years, and a mentor to others, in addition to his various customer and industry interactions. He thanks Joe for his contributions and hands him a gift. Joe opens the package—a bottle of Jack Daniel's, Joe's favorite!

Joe holds the bottle up in the air and gets a lot of laughs when he says, "Thanks Chris. I don't know if I'll be allowed to have this, right Lynn? But what she doesn't know about, she can't stop."

Next, Mike tells stories about sitting in the office next to Joe and the items Joe has in his office that attract colleagues to stop in, including the "golf ball in the water globe" brain teaser. Mike and Joe exchange barbs about who is the best at the water globe trick. Joe teases that the reason Mike is so good at it is that he "never does any work," which elicits more chuckles. Another is a stress-relief toy on a suction cup attached to his file cabinet, and of course the candy jar he kept filled with mints.

Mike then hands Joe a gift: the same type of water globe puzzle that they were just joking about. Mike demonstrates how to put the golf ball on the tee in record time before the globe is passed from table to table for others to try.

But Mike isn't finished yet. He then asks everyone to look at the business card next to their napkin. I didn't notice there was a card until he pointed it out. He asks if anyone sees anything unusual on their card and offers a prize to whoever guesses first. I study the card. It's a business card of Joe's with his picture on it. Looks okay to me. Mike prods everyone to look closely.

After a minute or so, a colleague of Joe's stands up and says, "Who is this on the business card? Kind of looks like Joe, maybe? He hands the card to Mike, who passes it to Joe. The card has Joe's picture and Richard Gere's picture as well. Ha ha, it's Gigolo Joe Gambill! The winner gets a box of candy, and Mike then tells the story of Gigolo Joe Gambill with a few embellishments and additional humor. When he's finished, he hands Joe another gift. It's an 8 x 10 framed "wanted" poster for Gigolo Joe Gambill, with a description of the character and a doctored photo of Joe on it. It's hilarious! The guests laugh as the framed poster is passed around the room.

As I look around the room, I see that the doorway is full of onlookers. They're golfer friends of Joe's who are playing today, and they heard about Joe's lunch. They're crashing the party to see Joe and be part of the fun. Next, Jean goes to the front of the room and picks up a gift. She hands it to Joe and describes a restaurant, D'Angelo's, that Mike, Joe, and others patronize regularly. The gift is a T-shirt from the restaurant for Joe to wear in Florida. Joe holds it up for all to see, and everyone applauds. Several of Joe's other colleagues thank Joe for helping them over the years, and they wish him well.

Now, Joe hadn't planned to give a speech, but he's caught up in the festivities, so he stands up and turns to face the group.

"Chris, Mike, Jean, and Jeanne," he says, nodding at each. "Thank you so much for putting this together. You've done a great job."

As he looks around the room, he tells the group how much working with them has meant to him. He says they're the brightest, hardest-working, and most enjoyable group he's worked with over the years. He says he hopes they'll visit him in Florida and that his home is

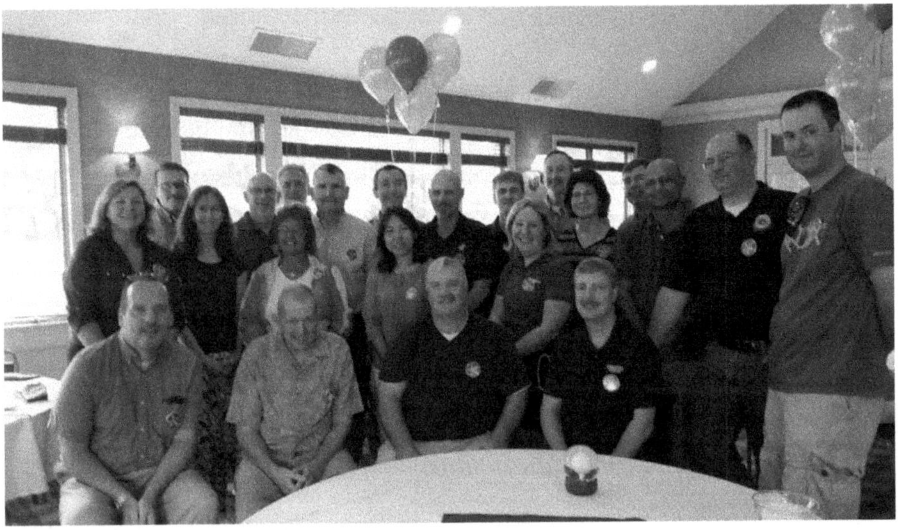

always open to them.

"This isn't the last time we'll see each other," he says.

He waves and sits down, and the crowd breaks into applause.

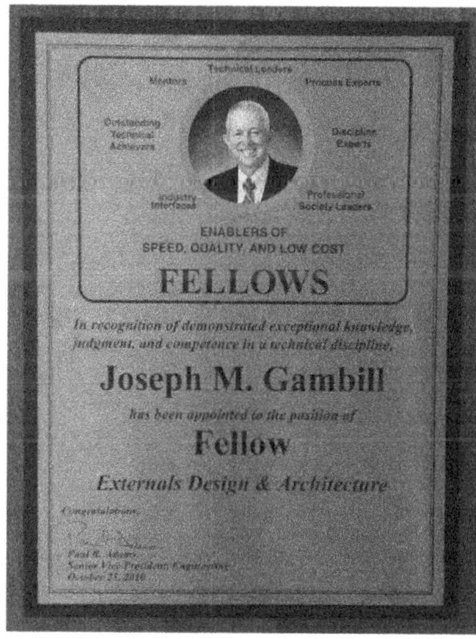

It was a wonderful event for Joe, and he thoroughly enjoyed it. As the guests leave, they approach Joe and talk to him one at a time. They exchange stories, and Joe asks them about how their families and work are going. A couple of them engage him in conservation with a technical question or two. Always engineers… and Joe humors them by either giving them an answer or directing them to where they can find one. The event lasts several hours, and I can see how tired Joe is. Jean and Jeanne are starting to pack things up, so I leave Joe with them while I bring the car around to pick up Joe and his gifts. Another trait of Joe's—he's *always* one of the last to leave a party.

◆

I drive home along the narrow winding hilly streets lined with colonial homes surrounded by summer green lawns with maple, poplar, birch, and red bud trees. Once we're home, Joe retires to the sunroom to read, but soon the book is resting on his stomach while his chest rises and falls with his quiet breathing. I use this opportunity to pack a few remaining items while I sit in the TV room connected to the sunroom.

The first item I bubble wrap and tape is Joe's Fellow of Systems Architecture and Design plaque. It's the highest technical achievement in our company: fewer than ten percent of the engineering team members are recipients. A review board evaluates and selects candidates for the award, and a dinner is held to honor the recipients. The plaque brings back memories of Joe's awards dinner in 2010.

> I'm wearing a maroon wool-blend suit and putting on a pair of single-strap black pumps with a low heel. Joe, usually ready before I am, is in the closet, deciding what to wear. He brings out a couple of suits and holds one up in each hand.
>
> "What do you think about wearing one of these?" he asks.
>
> "Well, they may be a little too big for me. Maybe for you though?" I respond. "Ha ha, you know what I meant," he smiles. "Should I wear a suit or a sports coat?"
>
> I walk to the closet and pick out a dark-gray suit. "How about this one?" I suggest.
>
> "The pants are too tight in the waist," he says. "This one?" He has a lighter-gray suit in this hand.
>
> "Yes, that'll look nice," I say.
>
> It's an unusual exchange, as Joe rarely asks my opinion on his clothing choices. He puts on his pants, though first he pretends that he misses putting his leg in one side of the pants, feigning to fall—always the joker. Next, he wants my opinion on his tie choice. Now I know how he must feel when I ask him about my clothes.
>
> "I think this red one will match," I reply.

"Are you sure—not too much of a power move?" he says, winking. He then selects a blue tie.

It's Wednesday night after work, and we came home to change clothes quickly before we drive to downtown Hartford. It's snowing lightly as Joe takes I-84W toward Hartford. It isn't that Joe is a bad driver—he's never even been in a car accident. It's the weather and the traffic that make me grip the car door handle tightly as Joe moves through the traffic. "Is that grip on the door you have making the drive any better?" he laughs, knowing I'm a nervous passenger and trying to get me to relax a little.

"Humph!" is my witty Neanderthal response.

We park across the street from the Wadsworth Museum and make our way past the closed ticket office on our right, up the stairs into the entryway. We aren't sure where to go at this point, so we follow familiar faces to the event setting. There's a string trio playing classical music, an open bar, and a gathering of colleagues at the event. We join the group and Joe exchanges congratulations with the seven other honorees.

We're just in time for the seating process to begin, and we're seated at one of twelve round tables. After our catered dinner and dessert, our company president and engineering senior vice president introduces the guest speaker: a retired female astronaut from NASA. After her speech, he then recognizes each honoree and invites them individually to the front of the room. Each recipient receives an engraved plaque, photographs are taken, and the dinner ends. For the next 30 minutes, more photographs are taken to commemorate the special evening.

◆

It's September 16, and we're leaving Connecticut on our one-way flight to Florida. Over the previous two weeks, the house packing was finished, Anthony and Al helped pack the portable moving container, the moving van picked up our furniture, the car transport company picked up the car, and the traveling veterinarian came to our house for a health check of the cats so Rascal and Simba can travel with us. There was so much activity as we were finalizing the move. Joe continued his at-home physical therapy with T, really looking forward to each session. He's had many visitors throughout this time as people wished him well. He was invited to lunch with his colleagues Mark and Dirk and had a good time seeing them. Joe is elated about finally moving and is feeling better every day since his time at St. Francis.

I'm on edge as Greg puts the suitcases in his car trunk. The much-anticipated moving day is here, and there are many logistics to manage. Joe is dressed and ready. We've had breakfast, using throwaway utensils and plates. Joe is having a little difficulty with today's schedule. He keeps thinking it's time to get in the car. Keeping exact track of time and plans is evasive for Joe, despite occupational and speech therapy over the months. With the excitement and last-minute preparations, the most important priority is keeping him comfortable.

This morning, I place the cat carriers on the floor and as each cat curiously peers in, I gently push them completely into the carrier and close the door. It's the surprised look in their eyes that tugs at my heart. I have betrayed their trust by closing them in. Now I open the carrier window, and in each cat's mouth, I put a pill that the vet gave us to reduce their anxiety when we travel. I walk through each room of the house, making sure we're leaving nothing behind. The new buyers purchased some of our furniture as part of the house sale, which allowed us to stay in the house until moving day. We're now ready to load into Greg's car—Greg in the driver's seat, Joe riding shotgun, and me in the backseat with the cat carricrs. I fccl no regret leaving the house for the last time as we head out for the airport. We have many good memories of living there, but it's also the house that Joe lived in throughout his diagnosis and surgery. I have such hope for our time in Florida and want to leave these difficult times behind—for a while, at least. Our decades-long "business trip" to the wintry state of Connecticut is finally over.

Chapter 7: Surprise

Because I could not stop for Death –
He kindly stopped for me –
The Carriage held but just Ourselves –
And Immortality.

Emily Dickinson

We move through the airport slowly on Friday morning, navigating the early chaos of business travelers in the morning and weekend vacationers later in the day. We manage regulation-size carry-on luggage and two soft-sided cat carriers while an airline employee tends to Joe in his wheelchair. We use electronic tickets and have our phones ready for each step of the security checkpoints. Once again, being pre-approved for expedited security helps considerably. The wheelchair attendant helps Joe's security check go fairly smoothly, but I'm required to take each cat out of his carrier and place the carriers on the belt for screening. I have to carry each cat with me separately as I'm checked. I choose Simba first, as I expect he'll be the more difficult one. Thank goodness I put harnesses and leashes on the cats for the trip. Simba is wiggling and meowing, so unhappy with the travel process. I hold tight to his harness to be sure he doesn't escape, talking to him in as soothing a voice as I can muster considering my own apprehension. One down; now it's Rascal's turn. He presses his body close to me as if to be shielded from the process with languid movements.

We sit at the airplane gate for an hour before boarding, with Joe leading the wheelchair brigade as Greg and I sit across from him. Boarding and takeoff are uneventful, except for the cats meowing loudly and trying to find more-comfortable positions in their carriers. We settle in for a relatively smooth three-hour flight. Our trial trip in June prepared us well. Our usual worries when we travel, such as renting a car or Joe using the bathroom, are significantly reduced because Greg is traveling with us. The drive to our new home is a blur in surreal time. The contrast with where we left is so sharp that it's almost unbelievable. So sunny, skies a completely clear azure blue, wisps of cloud trails as we travel north on I-95. The highway appears flat, light gray from the sun, and mostly straight. Traffic moves along freely at a nice pace for a Friday mid-afternoon. We're all smiles as we arrive at our new home.

Since the house is mostly furnished already, we adapt quickly to our new permanent surroundings. We adjust to the house layout and one-floor home easily. Joe starts new habits, replacing his prior sunroom favorite with the lanai and multi-windowed family room boasting lake views. Already Joe is reading the morning newspaper on the lanai. Each day we go for a walk, enjoying the warm weather yet careful not to become overheated as we become accustomed to the change in temperature. Our neighbors are friendly, and we meet them one by one when we take our daily walks.

Prior to Joe's diagnosis, and once we contracted to purchase the house, I talked to my sister Kathy about our plans for the new house. When I explained where we'd be moving, she told me she knew someone who was living in the same neighborhood.

"She's such a nice person," Kathy says. "Her name is Karen, and I've known her for years. We've crossed paths in our industry several times, and she works remotely at the same company I do."

It's a small world after all, I think to myself. What are the odds? We met Karen when we took our trial trip in June, and we immediately became friends.

Today, Karen stops by to see how we're doing and asks if she can do anything for us. It's such a help to get to know someone who's familiar with the area and gives us good advice on the basic logistics of our new environment. And so very thoughtful.

The driver of the portable moving container calls and asks to deliver the container earlier than planned. That means Greg will be here to help unload our boxes, a chore I wasn't looking forward to doing alone. Then the moving company calls and offers to deliver the small amount of furniture we shipped. And the car transporter does the same. I can't believe our good fortune: within a week, all our belongings from Connecticut are delivered. Seems like this move was meant to be.

◆

Before we moved, I asked our primary care doctor for a referral physician in our new area. Unfortunately, he didn't have any contacts in the area, so I tried to find referrals via our insurance company. That approach wasn't very fruitful, but I did some online research and found a well-rated primary care doctor in the area. I made appointments for Joe and me, but the soonest appointments available were in March—even after I explained Joe's medical history. So, I asked about an appointment with a physician's assistant and had better luck. I decided it would be a start at least and would establish us as regular patients with a doctor's office. Before we moved, I took Joe to his eye doctor and dentist so we'd have more time to establish patient-doctor relationships with them, also.

My parents, who've been steadfast in their long-distance support, drive to visit us the day after Greg returns to Connecticut. I know how fortunate I am to have my parents in my life, as they've provided a strong grounding base throughout Joe's illnesses. They love Joe and are devastated about his illness. I've learned, though I haven't accepted, that I can't overcome medical illnesses—at least Joe's. I can try to be as positive as I can and not transfer my worries to Joe, and we'll just enjoy our time together. My parents are problem solvers by nature and have many years of experience to bring to our situation.

While they're visiting, my father spends most of the day talking to Joe about sports, current events, entertainment, and what he and my mom do at their home. Joe and my dad have built a solid relationship over the 28 years we've been married, and they enjoy each other's perspectives even if they don't always share them. My mom helps me unpack glassware and arrange things in the china cabinet. Just having her near me is such a comfort. We try a couple of restaurants with them and start to get to know our new surroundings. Too quickly, their time with us is up. It's been great to have their company. We left Connecticut to be sure to avoid another deep-freeze winter, and we knew we'd be closer to my family for much-needed support.

My parents call me to let me know when they've arrived home safely, as we normally do when we travel. While I'm on the phone with them, I hear a garbled sound, almost guttural. I walk toward our bedroom door and see Joe sitting on the bed, his body taut and rigid. His chin is slightly up and his jaw appears locked. I hang up immediately and call 911.

I'm not sure what's happening, but I think Joe is having either a stroke or a seizure—neither of which I've ever seen firsthand. I check his mouth to be sure he hasn't locked his jaw on his tongue and see that he hasn't. (Truth be told, I'm not sure what I would've done if he had…I hadn't really thought that far.) He slowly starts to slide off the bed, his knees bent and his back pressed against the side of the bed, but there's no jerking, shaking motion. I talk to him constantly, telling him everything will be all right—hold on, hold on, help is coming, I love you, it'll be all right, I tell him over and over. He stops making the garbled sounds, but I wish they'd continue, because at least then I'd know he was trying to communicate. I feel useless not knowing what's happening and how to help.

The ambulance arrives quickly, as I see the red flashing lights passing through the stained-glass front door and reflecting on the living-room wall. I grab pillows from the bed and place them around Joe to keep him upright, and I race to the front door to unlock it. Three EMTs push a stretcher into the foyer and follow me to the bedroom. They pick Joe up, and he's less rigid now, which allows them to move him. They quickly look at his eyes as I explain the circumstances. They ask me how long he appeared to be rigid, and I'm caught off guard by the question—it hadn't occurred to me that it might be important. I give a best guess and tell them maybe five minutes.

They're wheeling the stretcher toward the front door as they ask me questions, and I'm walking fast to keep up with them. They tell me they're taking Joe to Tradition Medical Center, unless I prefer to go to the Martin Health System (now called Cleveland Clinic Martin Health), which is 30 minutes from our house. I opt for TMC. The EMTs ask me if I want to ride with Joe, but I decline because I know I'll need a car to return to the house to check on the cats. My next-door neighbor, who came outside when he saw the ambulance lights, offers to take me to the hospital. It's very kind of him, as we've only recently met, but again, I decline for the same reason.

I grab my belongings from the house and back my car out of the driveway, following the ambulance lights after they drive down the street cul-de-sac to turn around. I haven't been to the local hospital, and I have no idea how to get there. Clearly I wasn't prepared to, as I wasn't anticipating I'd need to know—certainly not this soon, anyway. A mistake on my part. Fortunately, I'm able to follow the flashing ambulance lights, and I find my way to a parking area in front of the hospital while the ambulance drives through an emergency entrance. The hospital appears to be under construction, and I can't find the hospital entrance easily. It's now about 9 p.m. Sunday, September 25. We've been in Florida nine days.

When I go to the emergency area, I find Joe resting on a stretcher that is one of several lined up in the emergency room corridor. What's this? I stand next to him and hold his right hand. He recognizes me, he can see me, and he asks me what happened. I tell him I don't know exactly and that we're in the hospital to try to find out, but that we're in good hands and will know soon. I spot an uninhabited stool on rollers and wheel it to Joe's bedside so I can sit next to him. He's breathing comfortably and has his eyes closed now.

I don't understand the apparent chaos in the emergency room. I spot a nurse's station and request that a nurse check on Joe. Soon after, a nurse checks his blood pressure and his oxygen level and fills out some paperwork after asking me questions about Joe. I ask the nurse why Joe is in the corridor, and she explains that a couple of patients are using the ER rooms because the hospital is at capacity. She tells me that's the reason the hospital is under construction. I'm a bit "assertive" at this point, advocating for Joe. Very tersely, I explain his medical history and his need for immediate attention. I insist that a doctor needs to see him quickly and that he needs to be moved from the corridor into a quieter area. Nothing happens right away, but the squeaky wheel gets the grease…and at this point, I'm very squeaky.

◆

Joe has been moved from the corridor to an ER patient room. The ER doctor orders a CT scan and X-ray. Based on the findings, an MRI with and without contrast* is scheduled. The results of the CT scan and X-ray indicate Joe experienced a seizure, but that's basically all we know at this point. We're told Joe will be admitted to the hospital when a room is available and will be relocated as soon as possible. Since the seizure, Joe is fatigued but is responsive. He understands where he is, what time and day it is, and that I'm with him.

He falls in and out of sleep throughout the night and isn't intimidated by being in an unfamiliar hospital. He knows he's had a seizure and tells me he was able to hear and comprehend everything going on around him while he was having the seizure. He explains that he listened to my voice, understood what I was telling him, and was comforted knowing he was being cared for. The garbled sound I heard from him was the result of his effort to speak. That surprises me, as I assumed he couldn't hear a word I said, much less remember what happened in so much detail. I had no idea that someone could be so aware while having a seizure.

Joe is receiving fluids through an IV inserted into his left arm. We can hear the activity in the ER corridors as there continues to be a lineup of patient beds, with nurses and orderlies busy helping others. Joe is in a much better location, although it's less than ideal. The ER quiets down by around 4 a.m. Joe is sleeping, but I gently wake him and tell him

I'm going home to change clothes and take care of the cats. He nods and then drifts off to sleep again.

Disoriented, fatigued, frightened for Joe, I try to remember where I parked the car. I thank God the car arrived from Connecticut earlier than scheduled. Once again, I chide myself for not preparing for something like this. Joe seemed to recover so quickly from his intestinal surgery. It seemed like we were back on track and our move to Florida went so very smoothly. Joe didn't need to actually participate in the move, but he seemed to handle it well. But now I wonder if the move was stressful for him and may have contributed to his seizure. I don't know for sure, but I'm so worried.

I don't know how to find my way home, and the car navigation system doesn't recognize the street we live on. It's pitch black, with a sliver of the moon providing minimal light. I try my best to retrace the drive to the hospital, and after a few wrong turns, I eventually find the way home. I feel completely drained as I collapse on the bed. A few minutes turns into a couple of hours, and I anxiously wake up, feed the cats, shower, and change clothes. It's light out now, so it's easier to find my way back to the hospital.

Joe is asleep in the ER when I return. It appears as if nothing has changed since I left, although the hallway is no longer full of patient hospital beds. I ask at the nurse station and am told no doctors have stopped by while I was away. I also learn there are still no hospital rooms available for Joe to move to.

◆

At 2:30 p.m. on Monday, Joe is taken to get the MRI while I wait in the ER. It takes a couple of hours, so I pace the ER for a while before I walk around the hospital searching for a chapel, but I can't find it. I call Greg, Joe's siblings, and my parents to let them know Joe had a seizure. I don't think anyone fully appreciates the significance of what has happened, except for Greg. He understands and says he'll fly down as soon as possible.

The stark contrast of the clear, warm, breezy Florida day with the grimness of the hospital hits me as I walk outside. I try to think positive thoughts. It could be worse—we could still be in Connecticut. Already the low temperature is in the 40s. We're scheduled to fly to Boston for Joe's immunotherapy treatment tomorrow, but it's extremely unlikely now. Based on our experience after his surgery at St. Francis, missing another immunotherapy session will most likely mean he won't be able to continue participating in the clinical trial. What will we do now, I wonder? What options are available to help Joe? I try not to despair, and I pray for the best. We don't know this hospital or the doctors who practice here, and we haven't yet established an ongoing patient-doctor relationship with them in a way that we wanted to. Those concerns add to our level of discomfort.

I return to Joe's room, but I find someone else there instead. I quietly back out of the doorway, trying not to be too invasive. Before I panic, I ask a nurse where to find Joe and learn he's been assigned a room on the top floor, where he'll be taken after his MRI. I find my way to the stairs and walk up the six flights to Joe's room, planning to wait there until he returns.

The single room is quite nice, with an attached bathroom and clean engineered-hardwood floors. It seems to be a theme, as St. Francis had similar floors. I peer out the windows that overlook the parking lot, searching for a familiar landmark. I don't know which direction we live in, but I can see several intersecting roads in the distance. Joe is returned to his room close to 5 p.m. We didn't know about the timing of the MRI, and Joe hadn't taken the prescribed sedative to help him relax. Between that and the seizure itself, he's quite tired when he comes to the room. The nurse assistant brings him a tray of food, and a doctor stops by to introduce himself while Joe is eating. The doctor, Dr. "S," explains that he's the neurologist who'll be reviewing the results of Joe's MRI. He asks several questions about Joe's medical history and completes a clinical evaluation of his current condition. He notes that Joe's left side is weaker than his right, which he says is most likely because of the seizure, and tells us he'll request a physical therapist to evaluate him. Lastly, he adds that Joe doesn't seem disoriented or impaired in any way but may feel more fatigued than he did before the seizure.

After Dr. S leaves, Joe and I agree that we both like him and feel that Joe is in good hands. I use my tablet computer to see what I can find out about his credentials, and I learn that he attended a top-rated university and had residencies at well-known and established hospitals in the U.S. Joe and I find this reassuring.

Joe ate a healthy portion of the hospital meal and is now fast asleep. At around 8 p.m., I'm surprised to see Dr. S entering the room again. He sees that Joe is asleep and confirms that I have a signed permission form to receive medical information about him. He asks if I have any records from Joe's prior MRIs, and I grab the hard copies out of the briefcase I bring with me wherever I go, which I keep all his records in. Dr. S tells me that the results of today's MRI is preliminary because they haven't been compared to Joe's previous MRIs yet but that he thinks it's best to share the findings immediately. My heart freezes and sinks when I hear that.

Dr. S tells me it appears that the resected tumor may be recurring. He tells me about the sizes and locations of various new lesions, but when

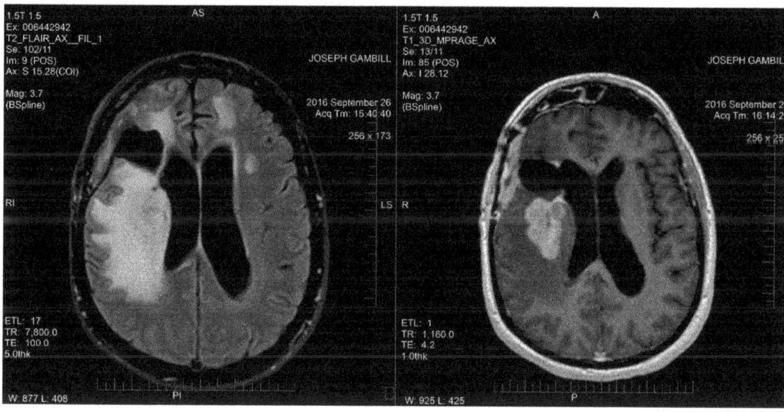

he sees I'm having difficulty grasping what he's saying, he suggests we go to the doctor's station so he can show me on the computer. I follow him down the brightly lit hospital corridor. It's so much quieter on this floor compared to the ER patient room. I feel as if there's no one else on the floor, even though I know there are patients in every room. Dr. S accesses various views from Joe's MRI files to explain the findings. In the first view, I can see the site of the original resection and a large darkened area that looks like it's attached to it. Dr. S explains that this is where he thinks the potential regrowth might be. He then shows a view of the left and right frontal lobes, followed by an area near the fourth ventricle. He explains that the brainstem is intact and that it's unusual for lesions to appear on the side of the brain opposite the initiation site. He's concerned that the glioma may have spread through spinal fluid and may have grown in his spinal column and elsewhere.* He says such a pattern of growth is unusual, although not unheard of, and that MRIs of Joe's cervical spine* and lumbar spine* may help determine whether that's the case.

Numbness envelops me as a I look at the results and listen to Dr. S's explanation. I automatically switch to a self-protection mode and ask him questions. Does the MRI explain the seizure? Will there be more seizures? Is surgery recommended? What about the clinical trial? What do we do next? I'm firing questions at a staccato tempo, trying to find answers that will offer solace, options, a different path. I'm totally reacting and not accepting what he's told me, searching for other possible explanations. Dr. S is very patient with me as he answers my questions. "Yes, this lesion in particular is in an area that could explain the seizure," he says as he points to the computer screen. He tells me he'll bring a seizure expert on to the case who can use an EEG to check the electrical activity in Joe's brain, possibly identifying the risk for future seizures.* He says there are also medications that can help control seizures.

Dr. S says that he's not familiar with the clinical trial Joe's been participating in and that I should consult with his doctors at MGH about the trial. He recommends against another surgical resection because it could affect his motor control and reduce his quality of life. Finally, he says he'll refer me to a radiation oncologist to discuss the treatment options.

At this point I explain that Joe has an appointment with Dr. P, who'll be Joe's local doctor if he needs one. I ask Dr. S if he's acquainted with him.

"Ah, yes, I've worked many patient cases with him," Dr. S replies, smiling. "He's an excellent physician."

We walk along the corridors to Joe's room. The hallway doesn't seem so brightly lit anymore; everything has dimmed.

Joe is awake when we return to his room. Dr. S explains the MRI results to Joe, and I see his chest deflate as if the air were punched out of him. He listens attentively and asks questions about treatment options. Dr. S repeats what he discussed with me and tells us he'll confer with Dr. P. Once again, we're very lucky that some things are working out the way they are and the two doctors already have a working relationship.

After Dr. S leaves, Joe doesn't look at me but stares at the white hospital room wall in front of him. I take his hand and hold it tightly.

"We knew this might happen," Joe says. "Now we need to understand the treatment options. It's good news that the new lesions are so very small and that we understand why I had a seizure.

"We'll find a way forward and have many good times," he adds. "I love you and Greg, and we'll be together for some time to come."

Joe is actually comforting me as he talks. Ever so calm, not arguing with the findings, and accepting that a new path will be forged. I, on the other hand, am planning to get a second opinion from Dr. D and the rest of the team at MGH. I don't completely accept what we've been told—not yet, anyway.

The hospital is very quiet tonight. Usually there are so many foreign sounds that make sleep almost impossible, but now everything is unusually muffled. The night shift nurse checks on Joe periodically, and the biggest commotion is when Joe needs assistance with the IV pole so he can walk to the bathroom, When he needs that help, the nurse isn't as quick to respond as I'd like, so I advocate for a quicker response time. Other than that, the late hours are hushed, leaving too much time to think about Joe's test results. In Joe's room is a bench that can be converted into a single bed, so I lie there restlessly, trying to sleep.

We'll get a second opinion, but the MRI images I saw today were quite clear. And the possible regrowth is larger than the resected tumor. Plus, it's in another part of the brain. It's unimaginable that I could lose Joe.

We've known each other since our mid 20s, and our hearts and minds are intertwined. Just the thought of him not being with me starts a panicky and suffocating feeling. But I just can't think about it now—I have to focus on getting him treatment and helping him recover. I need to be sure he's getting his needs met day to day. I feel so fiercely protective of him, yet ignorant of how to go about keeping him safe. Apprehension, foreboding, and dread are my companions tonight, each staring intently at me. I am in their grasp.

In the cold light of day, cautious optimism envelops me. My shadow companions from the night before are in the background of my mind now, no longer controlling my thoughts. The hospital physician checked on Joe early this morning and a physical therapist is arriving shortly afterward. Dr. K, a neurologist with a specialty in neurophysiology, has scheduled an EEG for this afternoon. Joe eats an adequate breakfast, which helps him regain strength. He has no noticeable impairments from the seizure, although he asks me repeatedly about the timing of the visits and the testing. While the EEG test is being performed, I call MGH to tell Dr. D about the results of the MRI. He's not available, so I talk to his nurse assistant. I explain the results quickly, and she asks if I can send the MRI file. Fortunately, both hospitals use the same data systems, so I'm able to save precious time by having the file sent to MGH electronically instead of shipping a disc. She says she'll ask Dr. D to look at the file as soon as possible.

Dr. K says the results of the EEG are consistent with the history of Joe's glioma and don't indicate any other abnormalities. As a precaution, Joe is prescribed an anticonvulsant medicine to prevent seizures. Also, the physical therapist's review indicates weakness in Joe's left side that's consistent with Joe's history, and he outlines a recovery plan. He tested Joe's strength, balance, and hand-eye coordination and walked with him even with the IV pole. Always wanting to please, Joe does his very best, even though it's clear that he's fatigued from the seizure. We're told he'll gradually become stronger over the next couple of weeks. Plus, the additional MRIs show no new abnormalities—what good news!

But the news that Joe's glioma has progressed is a crushing blow—our expectations for our future did not include that happening now. Always trying to be optimistic, we were so hopeful that the immunotherapy treatment would be a home run and that Joe would be among the small percentage of patients who would enjoy several years without the disease progressing.* From a small waiting area in the lobby of the 6th floor, I conduct a conference call to update Joe's brother and sister while he's in the hospital. The discussion is rather one sided as I explain the results of the latest tests. Jim is very quick to ask what he can do, and he asks how Joe is handling everything. Both siblings say they'd like to see him, so we make tentative plans. The news comes as quite a blow to both of them, as they hadn't foreseen losing their brother so soon. I also share the news with Joe's friends and colleagues, some with a phone call and others via text. It's hard for me to think about contacting others when I'm in the midst of processing the latest information and focusing on determining the next treatment steps.

◆

Joe is discharged from TMC on Thursday, September 29. After four days in the hospital, he's ready to come home. He has prescription orders for physical therapy, the anticonvulsant to prevent seizures, and a type of antacid.* He also has an appointment with Dr. P on Friday afternoon. I get the car from the parking lot while Joe is being taken to the front entrance in the wheelchair. He's very tentative standing up from the wheelchair and then sitting down in the car. He's strong enough to manage, but very hesitant, as if he's unsure of his own capability. I know my way home and am accustomed to the area somewhat, but to Joe, it's all new. He compares the area to Connecticut, pointing out the newer construction versus the older graying buildings we left behind. Planted flowers in vivid reds and purples are blooming in the median, and viridescent St. Augustine grass lines the sidewalks.

"I'm so happy we're in Florida. Look at all this!" he says, gesturing toward it with his right hand. "It must be starting to get colder in Connecticut, and we don't have to be there this winter. I don't miss that at all!"

Logistics with Joe are different since his seizure. He's using his walker again, and getting in and out of the car is more difficult. His thigh muscles are weaker, which is part physical and part psychological: he's overly cautious because he's not confident about his current capabilities. Sometimes being too hesitant can cause even more problems. I assure him that he's doing better, but I support him using the walker. Joe appears to be depressed with the latest news—who wouldn't be? But he isn't talking about it much.

Once Joe is home from the hospital, he keeps himself busy researching treatment choices online. There isn't too much new, it appears, but we'll wait until we meet with Dr. P tomorrow. Greg calls to talk to him, and they have a light conversation with lots of joking. In bed Thursday night, as I lie on my side pressed next to Joe's side with my arm across his chest, he reaches for my hand and holds it in his. We're both silent as we hold our thoughts inside. I'm reassured that Joe is with me, always a comfort, always steadfast. Our breathing is synchronized, and we gradually fall asleep together.

◆

We program the address to Dr. P's office into the car navigation system, and we're driving on unfamiliar roads except for I-95. We take exit 110, go east to US 1, turn right to go south, and turn left into a parking lot surrounded by what looks like a small outdoor L-shaped strip mall. "This can't be right," I think to myself before I say it out loud. I drive slowly past the yellow structure, reading each placard, and I notice that each one is medically associated. There it is—the sign with Dr. P's name. Well, I guess this is it, but it seems very unusual to me. It's too hot to leave Joe in the car for more than a minute or so, but I walk to the front door of the "office" and open it. Okay, it appears to be a legitimate doctor's office, so I walk to the car and help Joe out after I set up his walker.

Once we've checked in and are seated, I still feel uneasy and decide to talk to the receptionist a bit. I learn that the entire outdoor mall is used for various medical practices and that the radiation equipment is next to the doctor's office area. The building was used originally for retail stores, then restaurants, and now medical practices. It's very close to the Martin Health System, which is one of the locations the doctors are affiliated with. Still strikes me as odd.

We wait a few minutes, as is typical at a doctor's office, and then we're called to sit in a different waiting room. We know the drill, so we take the appropriate seats and wait patiently. A nurse comes in to check Joe's blood pressure and temperature and asks us the purpose of our visit. Joe and I tell her what our original plan was—to establish a relationship between Joe and a local doctor in case one is needed at some point—but we explain that Joe's seizure changed that. We explain that we're seeking the doctor's recommendation for treatment based on Joe's latest MRI.

After ten minutes or so, Dr. P, a suntanned man dressed in the standard white doctor's coat, enters the room. In my mind, I sometimes associate a person's face with an animal when I first meet them. Dr. P reminds me of Smokey, the Bluetick Coonhound who's the University of Tennessee mascot. Dr. P has a longish face with slightly puffy cheeks, like Smokey's jowls, and his eyes are spaced symmetrically in his somewhat narrow face. His dark-brown eyes are surrounded by laugh lines. He speaks with a strong Southern accent as he introduces himself in a drawn-syllable style. He has comfortable, warm mannerisms that create ease in an otherwise very stressful discussion. We review Joe's history with him and explain the latest turn of events.

Dr. P tells us that he's reviewed the results of Joe's latest MRI and that his observations are consistent with what Dr. S found. He conducts a clinical evaluation like the ones conducted at MGH, and he notes the weakness on Joe's left side and his essential tremor. Dr. P also asks questions about Joe's balance and has him stand on one leg at a time. Joe does so fairly well, but not with tremendous confidence. Dr. P says he doesn't recommend surgery at this point, and he talks about a chemotherapy medicine and a type of treatment called stereotactic body radiation therapy (SBRT). SBRT is a type of treatment that uses high doses of radiation on a precise area. It sounds similar to the treatment Joe received at MGH that involved a mask being designed specifically for him.

Joe is keenly interested in Dr. P's recommendation and says he'd like to pursue the treatment. I ask questions about the timing for the start of the SBRT and chemotherapy treatment, and about getting insurance approvals. The doctor answers all our questions and explains that he'll refer us to Dr. R, who'll be handling his chemotherapy treatment. A nurse steps in at this point and asks Dr. P to step out for a minute to take an important phone call. When he does, I step out of the room also, to look for the bathroom. The nurse stays with Joe. We both return to the room at the same time, and Dr. P's eyes look at me quite directly as his expression softens a bit.

"Mrs. Gambill, you and your husband seem to have a pretty good understanding of the illness your husband has," he says. "I want to be sure you understand what this MRI means. The original tumor has continued to grow, and it's quite large. And based on the MRI history, it has grown very quickly.

"Radiation might help but we need to be cautious to avoid serious side effects, but we'll try," he adds. "And SBRT may help prevent growth of new smaller tumors."

Dr. P tells me he wants to explain it again to make sure I understand it clearly.

"Because the tumors are now in both sides of the brain, it's likely that spreading will continue," he says. "Are you sure you want to proceed with the treatment?"

I'm quite surprised by this conversation, as I really hadn't thought about it that way and Joe and I haven't talked about the possibility of spreading continuing.

"How likely is it to continue to spread?" I ask cautiously, trying to process what he's saying.

He looks at me as if I'm not understanding what he's saying.

"It's already spreading," he says, "and it will continue to spread."

I ask him how fast he thinks it might spread, but he seems to avoid being specific until I plead for a more definitive answer. He hesitates, pausing to think before he responds.

"I believe your husband has maybe three months without treatment," Dr. P says. "The treatment might give him another month on top of that, perhaps." He also reminds me that the prognosis isn't exact but that it's what he believes based on Joe's history and the results of the recent MRI.

Well, there it is—it's finally out there. I tell Dr. P that it's Joe's decision to continue treatment and that he understands the tradeoff between treatment and quality of life.

"Do you have any reason to think Joe can't make the decision for himself?" I ask Dr. P.

"No," he replies. "I just want to be sure you both understand the nature of the decision."

I thank him, and I mean it sincerely. We need to know what we're dealing with to make the best decisions we can.

Once we're both back in the patient room with Joe, we talk more about treatment. Joe wants to proceed, and so we will. Dr. P explains the next steps, including the schedules for having a mask made, SBRT treatment, and chemotherapy. The plan is to start SBRT in a week.

Overwhelmed by all the information Dr. P gave us today, I help Joe get from the doctor's office to the car, which is a bit more complex with the walker than without. It's still a beautiful, clear, sunny day, but my senses are immune to my surroundings. My feelings are turned inward—wrapped and muffled as if they're packaged in a large, soft cotton ball. I'm protecting myself from the information, deciding to focus exclusively on the near-term tasks that are necessary for Joe's care. It helps me feel I can control at least one thing when Joe's condition is so totally out of my control. I jabber as I drive us home, trying to be as positive as I can be.

"Wasn't Dr. P great?" I begin. "SBRT sounds like it will be the best plan. I'm so glad it's available. Good choice to continue treatment. It sounds a lot like what Dr. D at MGH outlined for us, especially the new chemotherapy treatment he recommended.

Fear, despair, and futility are circling me, so I push back by focusing on Joe's everyday care.

I feel it's my job to help Joe with the treatment that he wants to pursue and to support him emotionally and physically. We work well together and have a routine that we follow. Since Joe's seizure, he's weaker and needs more assistance with everyday activities like standing up from a chair, taking a shower, and getting dressed. I'm worried about his balance—not because he has fallen but because he's so cautious that I think he's unsure of himself. Joe's physical therapy in the home will start Monday. We accept Dr. P's recommendations, but I still want to talk to Dr. D—I haven't talked to him directly since Joe's seizure.

Dr. D from MGH calls me on Saturday morning as he's driving into Boston.

"I'm sorry it's taken me so long to call you back," he says. I've been talking with Dr. S to stay updated on Joe's condition. How's he doing since the seizure?"

I explain Joe's condition and the treatment Dr. P has recommended: SBRT and chemotherapy. He listens and thoughtfully reminds me of his meeting with us in June when he mentioned that a change could be necessary. I acknowledge that and ask him his opinion. He says he supports both therapies and suggests we do them locally, which I recognize as code for "Joe's participation in the clinical trial is over." So I ask him qucstions about other clinical trials that Joe might qualify for, and he says he doesn't know of any that MGH is participating in. I ask him about Duke University, but he says he doesn't know enough about their studies to recommend one but will find a point of contact there for me.

Dr. D has been a constant source of confidence for Joe and me, and I realize we'll no longer be dealing with him now that Joe is no longer in the clinical trial at MGH. I thank him for his treatment and support over the last several months. He wishes Joe the best of luck and tells me he's available for any other consultations if we need him. My heart is very heavy as we finish the call, knowing Joe is entering a phase of his illness that isn't likely to be effective. That's why Joe entered a clinical trial to begin with. Desperation and fear have a hold over me, and as much as I try, I can't shake them.

Joe and I continue our routine as if we haven't received the news about his treatment. But while Joe is napping in his chair after lunch, I make phone calls to Greg, Joe's siblings, my family, and Joe's closest friends and colleagues. I quietly explain the circumstances and let people know that Joe's time is shorter than we prayed for. I begin arranging visits with those who'd like to see Joe while he has the stamina to entertain guests. I also believe I shouldn't leave Joe alone, so I put together a calendar of visitors to stay with us so there are neither overlaps nor gaps with no visitors. Greg, Joe's siblings, my sisters, my parents, my nephews, and Joe's friends all want to come see him and spend time with him, so I'll coordinate their visits around his new treatment schedule.

My sister Peggy is the first visitor, arriving Sunday. From the front entryway brick path, I watch her approach the driveway in her huge SUV. When she steps down from the driver's seat, we give each other a hug. We're not a "huggy" family, but under the circumstances, it just feels right. We unload the SUV and bring her luggage into the bedroom she'll be staying in. Joe walks with his walker from the TV area to the front of the house to greet her. Peggy is quite good with small talk, and she chatters about her drive, the other drivers, and the weather. She sits with Joe on the sofa and talks to him about her husband and children, filling him in on the latest with jobs, golf, her children's dating statuses—general news. It's such a help to both of us for her to be here. And it's a distraction from the reality of Joe's illness. Peggy just watches and sees what needs to be done—like grocery shopping, cleaning up after we eat, laundry—and pitches in to help in any way she can. And she's easy to be with, never making demands or prioritizing what she wants over what Joe needs. She's planning to stay for a week and be with us at doctor visits and at-home therapy visits. Joe and I have been handling these things until now, so it's such a help to have Peggy participate with us and have a third opinion on the various types of care.

Joe has many things scheduled for the week. His first physical therapy appointment is scheduled for Monday, his first doctor appointment with the chemotherapy specialist is Tuesday, construction of the radiation mask on Thursday, and ongoing physical activities to help him regain his strength since the seizure. On Monday, we meet F, Joe's new physical therapist. To my surprise, I find out that he's the manager of the physical therapists with the company he works for. At first, I think it's great news. Then I find out that our insurance requires that physical therapy be provided by an RN, not an assistant—hence the manager. F's clearly very qualified, and he conducts a thorough evaluation and outlines an exercise regimen consistent with prior evaluations. Joe does what he always does when he meets someone new and starts searching for a connection point. But F is having none of this—he's all business and is impatient when Joe has trouble keeping up. I talk to him a little when I notice it, ensuring him that we'll work together outside of the actual therapy visits so Joe will improve quickly. I want the two of them to develop a rapport, as I know it'll be a major motivation for Joe. Twice-weekly physical therapy visits are scheduled, each for about an hour including the evaluation and some exercises. F suggests that Joe walk every day in addition to doing his exercises—twice a day, if possible.

Joe seems to be himself: he continues to enjoy company, understands his surroundings, and engages in all that's going on around him. But he's more tired than he was before the seizure. And more tentative about walking on his own, instead wanting to use his walker. F encouraged him to walk around the house without the walker and perhaps use it only when we take walks outside. When Peggy confirms with him that Joe can use a cane instead, she finds a medical store nearby and buys Joe a cane. She picks out a very special one: it's black, with cats on it. She ties a large red bow and hands it to him. Joe laughs when he sees it, and immediately the two of them start "practicing" to coordinate steps using the cane for support. It seems like just the right thing to use around the house.

◆

On Tuesday, the three of us drive to Fort Pierce for Joe's first appointment with Dr. R to discuss his chemotherapy. I checked Dr. R's credentials prior to Joe's appointment and learned he graduated from a well-known university in the Northeast and completed his residency in a prestigious cancer specialty hospital in New York. I'm comfortable with his medical background, although I'm not excited about an appointment in Fort Pierce. Fort Pierce has a reputation as being a bit rougher than other areas, so I'm apprehensive about the trip and what the office will be like. We don't know our way around the area, and each new place we go is a learning experience. The drive north on I-95 is uneventful except for having to navigate the traffic caused by two bridge construction sites with three lanes narrowing to two.

Once off the interstate, we head east to 25th Street, then find our way to a three-story white painted concrete medical facility. Thank goodness for navigation systems! We figure out where to park, the location of the entryway, and which floor to go to, and we take the elevator to the doctors' office. I'm used to waiting for doctors' appointments, as they're often behind schedule as the day progresses. There are more new patient forms to fill out, which bridges the gap between our appointment time and the actual time Joe is called in even though we've become quite expert at completing them. We have an entourage of three, and we follow the nurse through narrow corridors with several turns until we reach the patient room. We each take a seat and wait again—for 45 minutes longer.

Finally the door opens, and a balding man with dark hair, pale skin, and the standard white lab coat enters the room. He introduces himself and apologizes for the wait, explaining that he was on a conference call with Dr. P and Dr. S about Joe's history and current condition. Dr. R then explains that Joe's recent MRI was the principle discussion point, and he acknowledges Joe's history, recent visit with Dr. P, and choice to use SBRT plus chemotherapy as treatment. He sits across the room from the three of us on a black round stool with wheels.

Dr. R maintains eye contact with Joe as he begins to talk about chemotherapy treatment, explaining that the treatment would be administered twice a month at one of his office locations. He explains the side effects of the treatment, including fatigue, nausea, and hair loss. He asks Joe several times if he wants to undergo the treatment considering the advanced state of his condition. Each time, Joe clearly says he wants the treatment. The doctor does not appear to be happy about it, as if it may be ineffective and actually impact Joe's quality of life. But he acquiesces and agrees to Joe's wishes. I'm puzzled by this exchange, as I thought the doctors were aligned with the course of treatment. Better to try than to give up, as the alternative is something we can't accept.

As we leave the doctor's office, we hear conversation at the nurses' station about the weather. The administrative staff is discussing the possibility of a hurricane reaching the east coast in a couple of days. Whaaaat?! I have to admit that I haven't been paying much attention to the weather, as I feel like I'm already living with hurricane emotions swirling around inside me.

The first thing we do when we get home is check the weather report on TV, which basically supports the office chatter: a category 4 hurricane, Hurricane Matthew, is almost at Haiti and Cuba with predictions that it may come up either coast of Florida, but most likely the east coast. A category 4 hurricane may involve sustained winds from 130 to 150 mph and is considered a major storm. If a storm of this intensity passes over our home, we could expect to lose electricity for some amount of time and perhaps lose cell phone service. Not to mention wind, rain damage, and potential for flooding. We're not located right on the coast, but we're close enough to be quite concerned. And we don't know the area well enough to know what could happen if a storm surge backs water up inland. We decide we'll wait to hear the weather report on Wednesday to determine whether we'll stay or leave. I'm afraid to stay if it hits our area, because if Joe has another seizure or some other emergency, I may not be able to help him. On the other hand, I don't want to drive inland if we don't have to. If we wait too long to decide, the routes out of our area will quickly become congested.

At this point, with the recent news about Joe's condition, this is just another item to put on the list to worry about. In the meantime, we make sure we have water, canned goods, and batteries on hand. Joe has appointments later in the week to start making his radiation mask, and Dr. P's office calls us to let us know they may need to be postponed. We're all watching and waiting to see what Hurricane Matthew may do.

◆

It's Wednesday, October 5, and we've been in Florida for three weeks. The weather reports continue to predict Hurricane Matthew will hit our area as a category 4 or perhaps a category 3 storm. Either way, we decide it's best to leave the area. Peggy will return to the west coast of Florida and Joe and I will retreat to my parents' house in the middle of the state. Karen, my sister's friend who lives a couple of streets over from us, has continued to stop by often to spend time with Joe and me. She knows the area well and has been so helpful to us as newcomers to the region. We invite her to come with us, but she decides to stay in her home. She offers to check on our cats after the storm to be sure they're okay, which is a huge help, as they don't travel well in the car. They're terrified of any type of travel, and they pant and cry constantly. I don't want to put them through the drive, and I'll need to focus my energy on Joe. Our home is a newer home, built to the latest construction standards, and includes high-impact glass, a strong roof, and concrete walls. My main concern is a power outage and loss of cell phone communication if there's an emergency. I feel comfortable that the cats will be safe if they stay in the house.

We leave at 1 p.m. on Wednesday. There's a little wind in the area, but you wouldn't think there was an impending storm unless you were listening to the weather reports. We take I95-N and then go west on Route 60. The traffic is steady, but not bumper to bumper, although it's much heavier than typical. Some people who live in mandatory evacuation zones farther south are seeking refuge in the northern part of the state, Georgia, and South Carolina. Gas is in high demand, and many stations have already run out. Fortunately, I filled up my car on Tuesday, so it wasn't an issue for us. It takes us an hour or so longer than usual to get to my parents' house, but at least the trip was uneventful—the best kind of trip.

There's something so grounding about visiting my parents. Although they're quite elderly now, they're in reasonably good health and haven't changed at all in their perspectives. Also, they're living in the same house I grew up in. It's changed a bit, with expansion and a major remodel a few years back, but as we drive in, it looks the same. For me, it's such an emotional relief to be here. At least something hasn't changed much in the last year. My parents haven't seen Joe since his seizure, and I can see they're worried about his physical strength. He works hard to stand up from the passenger seat before he reaches for his walker, which I set up in haste. We quickly decide that Joe and I will stay on the first level of the house so he doesn't have to walk up and down the stairs.

Joe and my parents get along quite well, and although there's so much pressing on our minds, we have quite a nice dinner, with lots of joking and political discussions. There's the upcoming presidential election that we all share our thoughts on. After dinner, we retire to the TV room to watch my parents' current favorite show, "Blue Bloods." Joe and I have rarely watched the show, but Joe is seriously enjoying it tonight. The plot seems to have a strong sense of right and wrong, with a happy ending. I can understand why Joe would like it. After all, our lives are not exactly having the happy ending we expected.

Hurricane Matthew passed through the area we live on October 6 and 7. A mandatory evacuation was instituted on the 6th, and many people had problems leaving the area quickly because of the road congestion and limited fuel. We averted those issues by leaving a day earlier. We stayed with my parents for three nights, as there was a possibility the hurricane would loop back. Fortunately, it instead turned east as it approached our area. We were spared the highest winds that were predicted, with maximum wind speeds clocked at 74 mph to 95 mph. Karen visited our home and checked on our kitties, sending us photos of their playtime together. It was a good decision to leave them at home.

◆

On Sunday, October 9, we return to our home. I'm rejuvenated after staying at my home of yesteryear and spending time with my parents. The drive south is also uneventful, and we arrive to a home with power, wireless Internet, cell phone service, and enough bottled water to last us six months. And of course, some very happy kitties.

Joe's home physical and occupational therapy visits will resume and construction of his radiation mask will begin this week. The hurricane also changed our schedule for visitors, so we have a full house planned for the weekend. My sister Kathy, her husband, her ex-husband, and their children, along with Joe's sister and her husband, will be visiting with us. And a close friend of Joe's from South Florida will be spending Saturday with him to watch a much-anticipated college football game, which will kick off at 3:30 p.m. It's the annual competition between the University of Tennessee and their longtime rival, the University of Alabama, and Joe wouldn't miss it!

The week passes quickly with Joe's therapist and doctor office visits, and guests begin to arrive. With the nature of Joe's illness and knowing an approximate timeframe, relatives and friends want to see him while he's still himself. Joe always loves having people to the house, and he so appreciates visitors.

People assume that he'll stop being "Joe" at some point, so they want to enjoy some quality time with him while they can. My sister Kathy and her husband Greg are a great help while they visit. Kathy makes dinner when they stay with us, and Greg and Joe's brother-in-law Jim help me by hanging pictures in the house. They do a great job, and it makes the house look so much more like a home. I realize it's a welcome distraction, as it gives me something to think about besides Joe for a couple of hours. Kathy and Greg also brought a power-lift reclining chair for Joe to use, and it made such a difference to him. Joe's legs have become much weaker, making it increasingly difficult for him to stand and sit from a chair. I tell myself it's because of the seizure, but I know it's also from the tumor regrowth. I push this into the back of mind for another day. They also brought a portable tray for food to be served on so Joe can eat while he's sitting in the chair.

The house is filled with people talking about current and past events. When Kathy's ex-husband Al visits, many stories are told about family vacations when our children were younger. Al is quite personable and a skilled conversationalist. Although Al is no longer married to my sister, we continue to have contact with him at various family functions, as they shared parenthood of two children who are now adults.

Al is seated on the dark-green loveseat from our prior residence, his left arm stretched onto the back of the cushion adjacent to him, his back to the water view. His oldest son, Chris, is seated next to him, and Andrew, his younger son, is on the couch facing the TV. Joe is slightly reclining in his new power-lift chair.

"Joe, you're looking good—much better than I was expecting," Al says in his heavy New York accent. "I mean that in a good way, you know. So glad to see you again. What's it been—six, seven years?

"How are you finding things in Florida? It must be much better than Connecticut, especially now," he continues. "I see the temperature is already getting frosty up north. You must be really enjoying it here. Weren't we lucky we dodged the hurricane? I had to evacuate from South Florida—so many people behind me on the interstate, and I got out ahead of the crowd. Had a little vacation, then returned home to no real issues. I can see things are pretty good around here."

He takes a breath, and Joe gets a word in.

"Yes, it's really great to be here," he says. "I can have my breakfast on the lanai, walk around a little bit outside, and yes, we were lucky with the hurricane."

Al says, "Well, I hope to see you in South Florida soon. We could take my boat out and enjoy some time on the water. Hey, reminds me of our summer vacations at Lake Placid. Joe, you were one mean jet ski driver, and the kids loved it when you took them tubing. They were always begging you, 'Uncle Joe, when will you take us tubing?' He laughs, and Andrew pipes in with a story of his own.

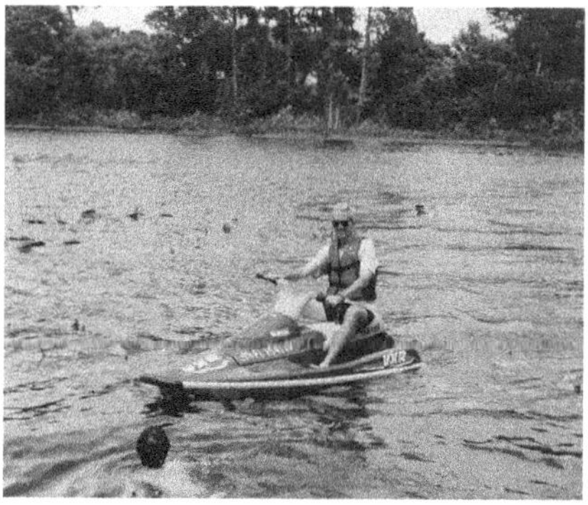

"Yeah, Uncle Joe, you were my favorite driver," Andrew says. "Except when you pulled Greg and me together—then it wasn't so great. Remember when our tubes hit and Greg and my heads bumped? Wow, that really hurt!

"And we really had to watch out for the weeds in the lake," he adds. "You seemed to have a great time pulling us through the weeds or driving around in circles to see if we could hold on. There was no way I was letting go when you drove through that!"

Joe smiles innocently. "Did I do that? Oh come on, I would never do something like that!"

Then the golf stories start, with recollections about playing the Lake Placid Golf and Country Club golf course for $15 a round.

"That course wasn't too bad," Al reminisces. "You couldn't beat the price, I tell you. And we had a great time playing with Bunker Bob and Mike. Bob was always in a sand trap, but he was really good at getting out of them. Those were fun times, weren't they?"

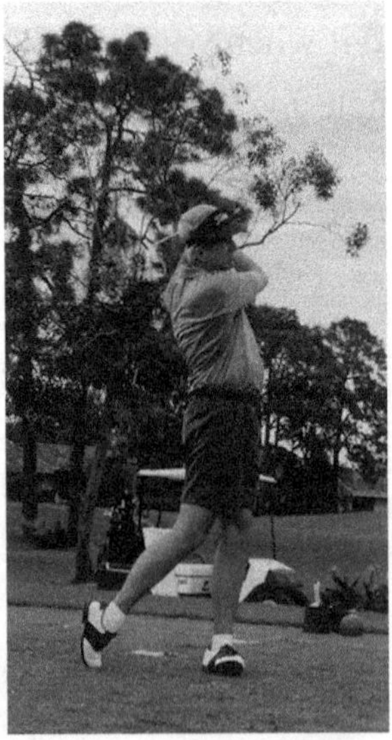

Joe smiles and nods in agreement. They're clearly reconnecting and having a good time. The conversation shifts to current events, the local area, our recent move—anything except medical discussions. But it's obvious from all the laughs and smiles that there's a close bond among all of us.

I'm walking back and forth, supervising the picture hanging and half listening to the conversation coming from the TV room. It's obvious that Joe is enjoying Al's company, as they always laughed together about whatever they were doing—boating, skiing, playing golf, cooking out, or occasionally jogging together. They have very different views on many subjects, but it never mattered, as they shared a common in-law family that drew them together on holiday events. Both are engineers by trade, and they share the talent for mechanical thinking. Joe would often follow Al to his garage, and before you knew it, they would be putting something together for the boat or the golf bag pull cart or something around the lake house—you know, the things men typically bond over.

Al understands Joe's health situation pretty well, as he dated a woman for many years who passed away from cancer. He was with her throughout her treatment and stayed by her side until the end. I'm in the den, looking at the pictures and other framed items that my brothers-in-law Greg and Jim hung for me—of Joe and his highest achieved awards, of our son Greg, and a few awards from my career.

Al walks in and says in says in his New York accent, "Hey Lynn, how are youse doing? This is a pretty tough time for all of youse. I know because my girlfriend passed away a couple of years ago, and it was the most difficult time of my life. To be with someone as they're fighting to overcome an illness that can't be beat and to watch as they slowly lose the battle—well, there's nothing I can say to make it easier.

But I can tell you that you have to be sure to take care of yourself along the way. The worry, the stress, the lack of being able to help stop the disease—before you know it, you're sick too. These hospitals are full of stuff—you need to watch out for yourself, too.

"Have you talked to anyone about how you're feeling?" he continues. "Well, I can tell you from my experience that it really helped me. There are people trained in how to help people like us deal with these situations, and they can help you. I mean, if you want the help, that is. I'm not trying to tell you what to do, just passing along what helped me. You'll be needing help from a hospice facility at some point, and they have some pretty good help there, as well as private specialists."*

When he takes a breath, I get a chance to say, "I haven't even given it much thought. You know, I'm consumed with taking care of Joe every day, and I feel like I'm getting good support from all of you."

I tell Al that I'll think about it and check with my insurance about what my plan will cover.

"Thanks for talking to me," I add. "That must've been such a hard time for you, and I'm sorry I didn't know sooner about what you were going through. We kind of lost touch, didn't we?"

About this time, I see Joe walking slowly, using the cane Peggy bought him, approaching the den to check out the pictures. Always with the quick words as he looks around, "Kind of a shrine to us, don't you think?" He winks as he says it.

"Love the pictures of Greg, they're great," he says.

He starts to sit down, using his cane for support, reaching backward with his left hand for the sofa. He almost misses the sofa, so Al and I reach quickly for him and help him settle onto a cushion. It's the first time something like that has happened, and I'm quite startled. If we weren't here with him, I think he would've fallen. It wasn't so much a balance problem as a leg weakness issue, I think. It shakes me up quite a bit, because up until now, I've felt like I can manage Joe's physical needs. I start worrying about him losing his balance as he walks, maybe having a problem in the shower, and then what would I do?

The weekend goes by so quickly, and our guests leave early in the week. Joe's SBRT treatment is starting on Thursday, with a total of five treatments planned—one this week and four next week. Then chemotherapy will begin on a two-week schedule. Physical therapy and occupational therapy continue twice a week. The occupational therapist listens when I describe Joe's near mishap over the weekend and decides to order a nurse's aid to help with his showers. We add a chair and hand railings in the shower, which will greatly reduce his likelihood of falling in the bathroom shower.

◆

Joe's brother and his wife, Jim and Allison, are visiting us for a long weekend, and I'm looking forward to seeing them. They arrive the afternoon of the day Joe has his first SBRT treatment. Joe describes his treatment to them after they arrive. He explains that he wears a new mesh mask that's fitted to his head and bolted to a table, much like the treatment at MGH. He says the radiation beam is directed to follow the perimeter of the tumor to kill cancer cells and prevent regrowth. The process takes about 45 minutes, during which time he can't move, he adds.

"My back is a little stiff when it's over, but they're pretty good at making sure I'm comfortable. One down and four more to go!" he says, smiling.

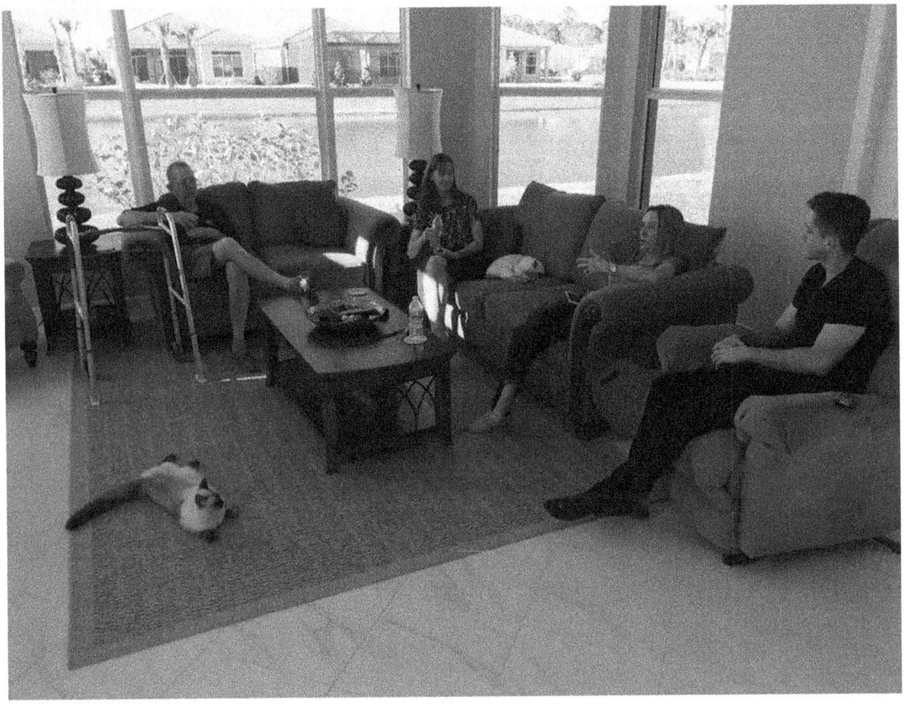

Jim and Allison are easy guests when they visit—they go with the flow, and they help however they can. We order food from restaurants for dinner and have standard breakfast and lunch fare. We go for walks with Joe while they're here, which are quite shortened since Joe's seizure. Jim keeps an eye on Joe so he's always ready to offer him help if he needs it—for example, getting his walker quickly if Joe decides to stand up and watching to make sure he doesn't lose his balance. Their visit is about spending time with Joe, talking to him, reminiscing, and enjoying some laughs. Joe is insistent about showing them around our new living environment so we go to the clubhouse and gym so Joe can show off a bit. Joe is more tired than the last time Jim and Allison saw him, and they're considerate of his current lack of strength.

Jim and Allison are preparing to take another ex-pat job, this time in England, and they're busy looking at rental real estate near their new office location. It's fun for us to be part of the excitement, and they show us many of the locations they're considering on the Internet. Many of the possible rental properties can be viewed online, so Jim connects his laptop to be viewed on our TV and the four of us discuss the pros and cons of various houses and townhomes. Moving to another country is such an adventure and requires a great deal of planning and consideration. The housing comparison to the US style is interesting and we all practice British accents and say things like, "Oh, now this is such a posh home—do you think they'll rent to a Yank? Reaaaaly?"

After Jim and Allison's visit, Joe has his last four SBRT treatments—two targeted to smaller tumors on the left side of his brain and the last two to the new growth from the original tumor resection site. One of the side effects of radiation treatment is fatigue. Joe didn't experience much fatigue during the radiation treatment at MGH; it seemed to come on after the treatment was finished. This time, he's showing fatigue after his first SBRT treatment. It may be because he also had a seizure, which certainly sapped his strength, but his fatigue from the radiation is noticeable early on in the treatment.

Although Joe continues with in-home physical and occupational therapy, it's clearly difficult for him. He tries so hard to please F and has improved, but he hasn't returned to his level of strength before the seizure. Every time we see F, he loosens up more. I chatter about everything I can think of, and Joe continues to joke with him. We now know a little about F's family, how things are at work, and more about his interests outside of work. He's a pretty good guy, and Joe and he are finally working well together.

◆

I'm constantly worried about Joe and won't leave him in the house alone since his seizure. I bought him a wheelchair, as his interest in walking outside has greatly diminished. I think it's important for him to leave the house every day for some reason or another—to go to a doctor appointment, the grocery store, the golf course or beach, or to go for a walk. Joe is fine with it, as he recognizes that his stamina is lower than before and he readily accepts the use of a wheelchair outside. I also purchased a baby monitor that has visual and sound capability, so if I need to go into another room, I can see Joe at all times. If he wants to get up and go to the bathroom, for example, I want to be there to help with the walker if he needs me to. He can do it himself, but I'm worried that he might lose his balance since he has less strength. He hasn't taken a fall of any kind since his diagnosis, but I've been very cautious since the incident in the den a week or so ago.

Karen stops by very early in the morning two or three times a week, bringing her work laptop with her. She visits with Joe while I go to the pool and swim a little to reduce my stress and help me gain perspective. Exercise has long been my go-to therapy to help me see things more clearly and get the benefits of a healthy activity. I easily lose my perspective as I continue to search for a path to divert the oncoming heartbreak for Joe. For the first time since his illness, I feel resentment building in me about his circumstances. I know it's a total waste of energy, but accepting the situation means accepting that I'm going to lose Joe. And I can't face that. I want to blame someone or something for it. If I take out my frustration, my despair assuming I can pinpoint the source, I can make it stop. I'm filled with emotional anguish thinking about losing Joe. Why haven't my countless prayers, novenas, and rosaries changed his path? Why aren't they being heard? Do we deserve this? Maybe I do, for some reason, but certainly not Joe!

Occasionally when I return from swimming, Joe has awakened and is sitting in his lift chair while Karen is working at the kitchen counter on her laptop. I often notice a little light banter as I walk in, and I can see they're becoming friends. Joe doesn't need a babysitter—he needs people around who care about him and can help if he needs something he can't get or do himself. Sometimes he's fast asleep and then wakes up shortly after I arrive. This morning, "me time" helps me so very much.

So many of Joe's friends want to visit him. Many don't understand the circumstances very well, so it's hard to explain that Joe's treatment and condition are slowing him down quite a bit. For example, going out to eat at this point is difficult. Joe struggles getting in and out of the car, and walking is a slow process for him, with or without a walker. He doesn't want to go out much at this point, except in the near vicinity. There's a lot of activity at the house now, with Joe's many visitors.

There's constant support from my family, with frequent visits from my parents and sisters. On the weekends, there are many more visitors. The last weekend in October, Bennett arranges for a few close friends to visit Joe and watch a University of Tennessee football game. Mike, who is Joe's friend from elementary school through college; Al, another college friend; and Joe's friends John, Stephanie, Paula and Jerry are arriving early evening to watch UT play South Carolina. Knowing that all these avid UT fans are going to make a lot of noise and that the game will likely continue past Joe's normal bedtime, I suggest that Joe take a nap in the afternoon, and he readily agrees.

While Joe is resting, I keep myself busy straightening the house. The camera monitor was moved into the bedroom in case I need to help Joe out of bed for any reason. Out of the periphery of my left eye, I see motion in the bedroom, so I glance at the nearby camera. Joe is starting to get out of bed, so I walk to the bedroom. But he must be half asleep—as he tries to stand from the bed, his legs slowly relax. He's sliding down the side of the bed, upright from the hip to shoulder, but his knees are bent. His eyes are open, but he appears groggy as I reach him. He's sitting on the floor his back leaning on the bed. He tries to stand, but his legs are too weak. I reach for the walker, pull it to him, and try to help him use the walker to pull himself up, but to no avail. I try pulling up on the back of his belt, but it's like pulling on a dead weight. I don't understand what's happening. Joe isn't having a stroke or a seizure, but his legs simply don't have the strength to lift himself up. I try to have him get on all four legs and then push from the floor up, but that doesn't work either. Then I call Karen, and fortunately she's home and comes over immediately.

Between the two of us, we're able to help Joe stand and use his walker to maneuver to the TV room. I ask Joe why he decided to get up without using his walker, which was next to the bed. He says he didn't think he needed it because he was just going to the bathroom. Well, a lesson learned by all, but I'm very worried. I realize that I can't get Joe up by myself if something like that happens again. And I can see that it's as if Joe "forgot" that he needed his walker while he was half asleep. I learned later that I could've called the fire department or EMT service for help. But I also realize that I'll need somebody strong to help me, as I can't manage by myself anymore.

I'm very preoccupied while our friends spend time with Joe watching the UT game. They very thoughtfully stopped by Duffy's and brought wings and side dishes to eat during the game and set everything up when they arrived. Joe sits in his lift chair while Mike, Al, Bennett, John, and Jerry crowd onto the sofa and loveseat. Stephanie, Paula, and I sit on barstools and talk about the usual things, such as our children and our interests. This is the first time Paula has seen Joe since his illness, as she and Jerry live in Alabama and aren't in our area very often. They made a special trip just to see him, because they understand how serious his illness is.

I think Paula notices how upset I am, and I finally explain what had happened in the afternoon. It's not quite the southern way to take it on directly, so Paula tells me about the death of her father, whom she was very close to. As she talks, I can see how it still affects her many years after his passing. She says she's so thankful for the time she had with him, even when he was too sick to really recognize her. She then reaches into her purse and gives me a small book. She tells me that her church prayer group has been praying for Joe and they wanted me to have the book, called "Jesus Calling" by Sarah Young. Her kind act all but unravels the calm front I'm trying to maintain. Another couple we've known over the years, Janet and Mike, live in the same town as Paula. Janet is part of the same church group, and I'm so very thankful for their thoughtfulness.

I can see Joe is enjoying himself, as he's surrounded by his friends of many years. I can also tell that he's much quieter than he would usually be as the group becomes more and more boisterous as the game continues. The usual yelling about various plays and colorful language are thrown around, all in good fun. Joe needs to get up to go to the bathroom, and I quickly get the walker for him. He makes jokes about how old he has become needing a walker. I see sympathetic looks for him as he walks to the bathroom, me next to him to help with his balance if needed. This is the one thing Joe didn't want: pity. But when you're healthy and see a close friend so very sick, how else can you feel? Maybe not pity, but sympathy? Wanting to spare your friend the changes you see are happening? Like so many things we're faced with that we can't change but have to accept and endure.

I don't think I've been successful in steering a shared evening emulating the past. There are too many changes in Joe for those who haven't seen him since his illness. I can see the caring and concerned glances Joe's friends make throughout the evening as they notice the changes in Joe. I know that Joe really is happy to be with his friends, and I marvel again at how he has continued so many friendships for decades. The camaraderie among the guests is genuine. It's a late evening for Joe, and our guests leave when the game ends. Bennett was so thoughtful to make the arrangements for this event, and Joe and I really appreciate it. I notice that Bennett is shaken by Joe's condition and is very worried as he leaves.

◆

The next weeks are filled with so many guests and visitors. Between Greg, my parents, my sisters, and Joe's brother, there are always two people in the house with Joe. At one point, my parents and my sister Peggy are visiting at the same time. I'm not sure what the best situation for Joe is as his illness progresses, and I start wondering if an assisted-living situation is an option. Peggy and I spend several days visiting many potential locations within a 50-mile radius of home. They each have their pros and cons, but the one thing I can't get away from is the thought of Joe actually spending his final days at any of them. They have various facades and offer care for Joe as his needs may evolve, but every one of them seems like such a very lonely place to be. After much soul searching, I conclude that it's not the best thing for him. He doesn't need that level of care yet, and I just can't let him spend his last days in an institution of any kind. So I'll be sure family and friends surround him, and if I need to hire any type of in-home help, I'll do it.

During this time, Joe started chemotherapy treatment, with an infusion every two weeks at Martin Health System in Stuart. It's quite different from the logistics of MGH, and I'm surprised at the setup. There are no private rooms, simply chairs lined up with patients receiving various infusion treatments. Some of the chairs overlook the beautiful St. Lucie River, while others face the inside of the infusion area. Once Joe is checked in and seated in a chair, we wait no more than ten minutes for the infusion to start. The nursing team performs no intermediary checks during the infusion process, and the infusion takes about 45 minutes from the time it starts. I assume that the differences are due to the protocol for clinical trial versus a standard chemotherapy treatment.

I've read that some infusion centers like to have patients together in a room when they receive their treatments as a way for them to feel less isolated and share the experience with others. I personally don't like it at all. It feels disorganized, impersonal, as if the nursing staff is doing something routine and ordinary. Maybe it's routine for the nursing team, but it sure isn't for us. When Joe's treatment is finished, he needs to use the bathroom. It's difficult for me to manage the heavy door and walk with Joe into the bathroom. Joe knows the treatment isn't very likely to make a difference to his tumor growth because of the type of tumor he has, but he believes that getting treatment is better than not getting treatment. He hasn't been especially impressed with the experience either.

As we drive home, Joe says, "I feel really tired, not like the infusion treatments. I'm going to rest a little on the way home. I'm just so tired…"

I keep glancing at him on the drive home. He's quiet and resting. I'm so glad we brought along a pillow so his head has some soft support.

Over the next four weeks, Joe has two more infusion treatments. Each experience is about the same, although we always try to establish rapport with his attending nurse. Before each treatment, we meet with Dr. R and he conducts a simple physical exam to confirm that Joe is okay to have the treatment. I ask him about Joe's fatigue, and he explains that it can be a side effect of the radiation and chemotherapy. Joe's left arm is showing signs of weakness, and his essential tremor is increasing, particularly as the day goes on. The weakness in his legs isn't improving, even with physical therapy. I observe these things and try to restrain my feelings of panic. I was so hoping the treatment would alleviate those symptoms and at least slow the progression of the disease, but I'm not sure anything is slowing down, except Joe's energy level.

Joe continues to have visitors constantly, and our house is always full of many well-wishers. Every day, there are cards in the mailbox for him, and he enjoys looking at them. The retired former president of the military engines division for our company and his wife visit Joe, which again speaks to Joe's reach with people and his exemplary work reputation. The two men talk about a particular tactical fighter engine that they helped design. Joe so appreciated this very special visit. Joe also enjoys visits by Brian, his nephew by marriage, accompanied by his wife; Al and his son Chris; and his friends Dan, Bennett, John.

Joe's brother visits for a week in November and once again is such a help. At this point, Joe continues to be fatigued from his treatments and rests more than he ever has. He's simply too tired to do many of his exercises, although he can walk around the house with his walker. We try to go for a walk outside every day, but now I usually end up pushing Joe in his wheelchair. Jim helps me take Joe to his final doctor appointment with Dr. P at Martin Health. Jim is so much stronger than I am, and he can easily handle Joe getting in and out of the car. Dr. P tells us that Joe's radiation is complete, and that going forward, Joe will see Dr. R, unless radiation is determined necessary in the future. Dr. P and Joe have a natural ease, and I can see that Joe is sorry to no longer be under his care. He was quite helpful to Joe by treating his tumors and preventing them from growing further.

Joe understands everything around him and participates in conversations, but it's clear that he's recognizing that he's becoming much weaker. I see the gradual change in him since the seizure, radiation, and first chemotherapy treatment. I'm frantic with worry internally, yet I try to hide it from Joe. Every night, I read to Joe from the prayer book Paula gave me, and Joe tells me it's been helping him. We start reciting prayers daily at the beginning of November, and Jim joins us for the prayers at Joe's bedtime every night.

As the end of the week nears, Greg joins us in Florida. Joe, Greg, and Jim have a couple of days together before Jim returns to work. The three men have so many mannerisms in common, and they share a quick, witty sense of humor. Together they talk about books they've read and movies they've seen, and they quote from each with amazing recall.

During this time, Joe tells me something's been on his mind—something he's been mulling over. He tells me he thinks he wasn't as kind to Jim as he could've been growing up, and he wants Jim to know he's sorry. He isn't sure exactly how to handle it, so I encourage him to talk to Jim while he's here. Direct, straightforward talk about his feelings usually isn't in Joe's wheelhouse, and I understand he's thinking about what to say to his brother. The last night Jim is with us, Joe asks him to talk. I don't know exactly how Joe talked to Jim, but they were together for quite a while. At some point much later, Jim tells me Joe apologized to him and they had a deep conversation and that he reassured Joe that he never felt Joe's concern was an issue growing up.

◆

Joe continues to want to try to do some things out of the house. Karen invited us to a party for her neighbors at the clubhouse, which Joe is adamant about attending. I have concerns about his stamina and I don't think it's a good idea to go, but he's insistent. Peggy is staying with us this week, and she helps me with the logistics of getting Joe in and out of the car. Joe is showing frustration about the help he's getting, even though he knows he needs it. He doesn't say it, but he shows his irritation by gently brushing Peggy or me away as we reach out to help him. It's a new behavior for Joe, as he's been taking things in stride up to this point. But when he tries to sit down in the car without help, he reaches for me and his eyes search my face for reassurance.

Once we're at the clubhouse, he enjoys talking to a few of our new neighbors as they make time to welcome us. It's clear to Karen's guests that Joe is very ill, and so many people just don't cope with sickness very well. We welcome Karen's kindness in inviting us, and we stay for about an hour before Joe indicates he'd like to leave. Joe made a commitment to Karen that he would go to her party, and he was determined to go no matter what.

Joe has started going to weekly Mass with me, at his request. We usually attend a Saturday afternoon service, and Joe and I sit at the rear of the church. Although Joe isn't Catholic, he tells me that attending

Mass is helping him and that he feels a part of the service with the warmth of the parish family. As Joe feels closer to his beliefs, I find that the resentment I'm developing is accompanied by burning anger for what is happening to Joe. It's been building up in me gradually, as I simply can't process what's going on. I can see the changes in him, yet I can feel him with me. His personality is changing a bit in that he's becoming more emotional, whether it be a reaction to a movie or an occasional display of frustration about his capability. I know that what I feel isn't logical, and perhaps it's even irrational. But seeing Joe gradually decline is shaking my faith. After so many prayers for him to be spared, why would God allow this to happen to him?

Joe's physical capability continues to decline ever so slowly. The shaking in his left hand is making it difficult for him to cut up his food. As I notice these things, I step in to help—for example, I now serve his food already cut up. Joe is struggling with these changes and it's very hard on him, yet he maintains his dignity. He jokes about needing help cutting up his food or using his walker. He's trying so hard to act like it isn't happening, but he knows it is. Despite seven weeks of treatment —one week of radiation and six weeks of chemotherapy—the disease is progressing.

We're hosting Thanksgiving this year, and my parents, Karen, Greg, and a couple of Greg's friends join us. Thanksgiving has been our family favorite holiday for many years, and this year, as hard as we try, the undercurrent of Joe's illness creates a somewhat false family happiness. On the one hand, I'm so thankful to be together; on the other hand, Joe's worsening condition is so very noticeable. He's been using his wheelchair to travel around the house—he uses his walker only occasionally, and he's set his cane aside. And now he's developed a new symptom that I don't know what to make of: once he goes to bed at night, he gets up every few hours to go to the bathroom. But he really doesn't need to use the restroom. It's like he's restless and wants an excuse to get out of bed. Because Joe retires earlier than I do, I use the monitor to watch for when he starts to get up, to be sure I'm with him. If I'm also in bed, I get up with him to be sure he uses his walker and doesn't lose his balance. He doesn't do it during the day, and I don't understand why it only happens at night. Thanksgiving is no exception.

For the first time since we've been married, I arranged to have a turkey dinner prepared for us rather than cooking the meal. Greg and his friends Colin and Annie cook their own vegan food, which generates delicious smells that fill the house. We sit together in the dining room for a family Thanksgiving, and my father says grace before we eat—not the standard "Bless us, oh Lord, for these thy gifts…" but his own words: "Today we celebrate Thanksgiving as a family, and we thank you, Lord, for allowing us to be together. We thank you for this food we are about to eat and for the shared company of those with us today. Amen." Joe lifts his water glass and says, "Hear hear! I agree—happy Thanksgiving!" We each nod our heads and respond, "Happy Thanksgiving!"

The turkey, stuffing, gravy, green beans, mashed white and sweet potatoes—everything is delicious. We enjoy the comfortable silence that comes when diners enjoy well-prepared food and sound relationships. There's too much food, especially with all the desserts available—Joe's favorite pecan pie and pumpkin pie, with ice cream and fresh whipped cream as toppings. I'm entertained listening to stories Greg and Colin share about their many antics, whether they're about trips to the gym, racquetball, or their friends. Joe is quiet, listening to the conversation during the meal. Joe and Greg have a very close relationship, and Joe loves having Greg with us. Joe is observing Greg, paying attention to what he says and how he talks. His eyes become misty behind his glasses as he whispers to me that he's so happy to see that Greg is doing well.

The evening before Greg leaves to go back to work in Boston, and after his father has retired for the evening, Greg joins me in the TV room.

"Hey, Mom, how's it going with you?" he asks.

I suppose I'm looking a little ragged around the edges as I get up a lot during the night with Joe. I tell him that I'm fine and that I'm happy he was with us for Thanksgiving.

"Mom, I want to be with Dad from now on," Greg tells me. "I can see the changes in him since the last time I was home, and I want to be here to share what time he has with us. I know it's my first job since I graduated, but it really won't affect my career. Who would find fault with me for taking time from work to be with my father under the circumstances?"

Greg tells me he can find another job later if his current employer won't grant him a leave of absence, but that he's reasonably sure they'll allow it.

"What do you think?" he asks me.

"I think you'd be doing something that for the rest of your life you'll be glad you did," I reply. "We don't know how much time your dad has, but clearly, he's getting weaker. We both love you so much, and having you here will be a huge help to both of us."

I tell him how proud I am of him and how lucky I am that he cares so much, and I ask him what type of arrangements he would make.

"I can finish my current projects from here, and I think that if I'm back for a week, I could then move here for as long as I need to," he tells me.

The relief and comfort of having my immediate family together, the love for my son—so much emotion washes over me as I watch him talking. The most important thing to me has always been my family. I'm so fearful of breaking this unit apart, knowing I'm going to lose Joe. It's as if I'm losing my identity as I see Joe struggle, watching him lose ground slowly every day. I'm so thankful for what Greg is planning to do, but I also worry about him. It's a lot for him to take on, and I so wish I could ease the situation. The best thing I know to do is to encourage him to have his closest friends near him a lot. I'm sure he'll talk to them about how he feels in ways he won't with me, trying not to upset me. So I encourage him to invite any of his close friends to also be with us, like he did for Thanksgiving.

◆

The Monday after Thanksgiving, Joe has an appointment with Dr. R followed by a scheduled chemotherapy treatment late morning. Joe is very tired from the radiation and chemotherapy treatments and isn't exercising, reading, or enjoying many things at this point. I don't know what to do about it, and I really don't know if it's because of side effects from the treatment or because the treatment itself is simply not very beneficial. Joe and I drive to the hospital in Stuart, and once we're there, we manage to get from the car to the wheelchair and up the elevator to Dr. R's office. As is now routine, Dr. R asks Joe how he's doing and Joe responds, "I'm doing pretty well."

I mention that Joe is getting up two or three times a night and appears quite restless, almost as if it's a spontaneous reaction to something.*

The doctor asks Joe if he's feeling better or worse over the last several weeks, and Joe admits that he actually feels worse. When Dr. R asks Joe how he's spending his days, Joe shrugs and tells him he's been spending time with his friends and me, watching TV, and sleeping a lot because he's so tired most of the time. The doctor asks about his appetite, and that is the one thing that hasn't changed—Joe eats quite well and enjoys mealtimes.

Finally, the doctor gently asks Joe if he thinks he should continue with his treatments under the circumstances. We know Joe's cancer is very advanced and that the radiation and chemotherapy treatments were a long shot. Dr. R explains that it's a question of quality of life and that the options are to continue with treatments and keep feeling the same —perhaps even worse—or stop treatment completely. The decision is up to Joe and Dr. R. Joe spreads his hands out and quietly says he should probably stop the treatments based on how he's been feeling. His eyes lock with the doctor's, in a searching appeal. He's trying to decide what he should do and is trying to read the doctor's response, maybe expecting him to disagree. Dr. R nods, puts his hand on Joe's shoulder, and doesn't argue. He tells us that he'll have hospice contact us and that he'll cancel Joe's treatment for today. Joe has his answer. This is the last visit with Dr. R.

I'm shocked that Joe is no longer going to receive treatment, even though I agree that the treatments don't seem to be beneficial. As Joe and I drive home, I ask him what he feels. He looks at me sadly.

"It's all happening so fast, and I just don't feel well," he says. "I'm so tired all the time, and I just don't think the treatment is helping me. I don't know what to expect, but I want a little dignity with the time I have left—not be feeling like all I want to do is sleep."

He reaches out and holds my upper arm as I drive us home. I don't know what to say, and I'm not sure how I feel. Continuing with treatment is analogous to hope. Just the word "hospice" terrifies me. I think of it as a service for someone who's approaching death.* I glance at Joe and recognize that his decision is about making final preparations for his passing and trying to have some remaining good times with us. I'm not ready for Joe to leave. I can't be without him.

Once I'm home and Joe is sitting in his lift chair, he leans back and closes his eyes. Soon his breathing is slower, even, and deep. I call Greg from the living room to give him an update. He just left yesterday and plans to return this weekend, but I think he needs to know right away. Greg tells me he's not very surprised considering how tired Joe seemed at Thanksgiving. He says his employers agreed to let him work remotely and relocate to Florida to be with his father. I'm so relieved, but I'm also inwardly panicking about how quickly everything seems to be happening. I make a few other phone calls to Joe's family, my family, and a couple of Joe's close friends.

Later in the day, a representative from hospice calls and sets up an in-home evaluation to determine the level of care Joe will need. He and I have a quiet dinner together. His left hand is quite shaky, and his right hand shows a slight tremor. Although I cut up his food for him, Joe can feed himself and is quite insistent on doing everything he possibly can for himself. After we eat, we have an unusually direct conversation.

"Joe, is there anything you want to do, anyone you want to see in the near term?" I ask him. "I know you talked to your brother—is there anyone else you want me to call and ask them to visit?"

Joe shakes his head and says he talked to Jim and has talked to Greg.

"Greg will be here this weekend, and I can talk to him some more," he says. "Other than that, I've seen family and friends and feel caught up."

I ask him if he'd like to write a letter to anyone—something he'd like for them to read later—or if he wants to give anything in particular to anyone. Joe says no, that he just wants to be with Greg and me and let things play out. He tells me that he doesn't know what will happen to him over the next weeks but doesn't want to be a burden. I immediately assure him that he's not a burden and that we want to be with him and to help in any way we can.

Joe's greatest gifts are his intellect, his memory, his sense of humor, and his knack for building relationships. And of course his golf prowess. These skills are slowly being stripped from him, little by little. It's so hard to know what he's thinking anymore and how he's processing information. He's conversing, yet he's sleeping more and more. I'm starting to believe that we each experience our own form of purgatory and hell on earth before we leave this earth. Joe is in purgatory now, and he's approaching his time in hell on earth.

Chapter 8: Hospice Care and Disease Progression

Yea, though I walk through the valley of the shadow of death,
I will fear no evil: for thou art with me

Psalm 23

The incidence* of glioblastoma multiforme (GBM),* Joe's type of brain cancer, is two or three per 100,000 adults. GBM accounts for 52 percent of all primary brain tumors* and about 17 percent of all brain tumors (both primary and metastatic).* These tumors occur most often in adults between the ages of 45 and 70. By comparison, the incidence of lung cancer in the United States is about 24 times the incidence of GBM.

Because GBM is so rare and the causes (and so, prevention measures) unknown, there's a lack of information on the disease and what to expect, other than that death is certain. Also, the most appropriate care for a patient in an advanced stage is not well defined, as each patient's case is unique. I believe that if there were more research on GBM, the treatment, prevention, and overall experience of patients and their families would be greatly improved.

◆

By 28 days after Joe's treatment was stopped, he had progressed from feeding himself, talking, and walking to staying in bed full time. The changes we noticed included:

- Increased shaking in his left hand first, then in his right hand
- Difficulty walking: he veered sharply to the right
- Continued and increasing weakness in his thighs
- Increasing impulse to stand when seated—eventually, almost every fifteen minutes in the daytime and five times during the night
- Loss of bowel control
- Gradually reduced speaking ability, until he was unable to speak
- Inability to swallow

Joe is with either Greg or me at all times as his disease progresses. The hospice service evaluated his condition and determined a nurse would see Joe twice a week. Hospice also assisted with personal hygiene, initially with helping in the shower and eventually to bed baths as his risk for falling increased. The hospice staff shows me how to turn Joe from side to side and give him a bed bath. I shave him every day, as he's always so very fastidious about his appearance. He jokes and pretends that I cut him while I shave him, and he laughs and laughs about it. I also trim his hair, as his last professional haircut was just before Thanksgiving. He likes his hair short, which makes it easy to maintain.

Greg relocates shortly after Thanksgiving to be with us as his father progresses. When Greg arrives, Joe is using his walker less and his wheelchair more. We take short walks around the neighborhood, with

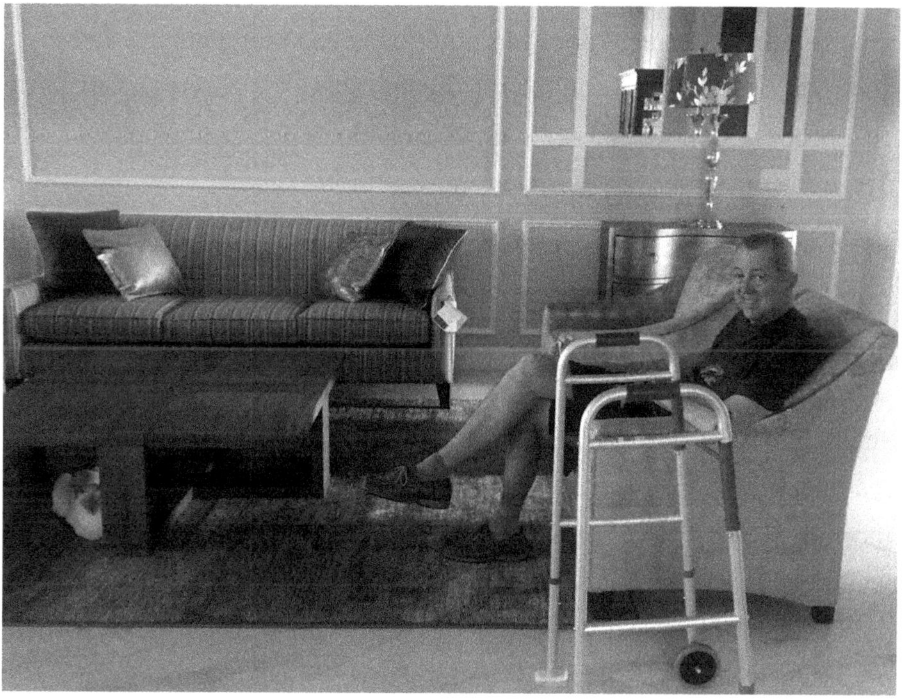

Joe in his wheelchair. We also learn to help him sit in his wheelchair by positioning his hands on the chair rails and then holding him under has arms to support him as he sits down. At first we can manage with only one of us helping him, but in a couple of weeks, it takes two of us to do it safely. Joe is frustrated that he needs help, and he wants to do it himself. He's especially concerned that he's losing control of his bowels. He's no stranger to that problem, as he had colitis, a form of irritable bowel disease (IBM), for many years before it was in remission.* But it's different this time: he has little warning, and he's gradually losing more and more control. We learn to adapt by having Joe wear protective underwear, although he absolutely hates it and repeatedly tells me it's totally undignified.

Hospice is a great help to us, offering not only nursing assistance but also some counseling and ministry support. We meet with a hospice social worker, who has a minister meet with Joe at our house. It's a time of severe distress for our family. Joe is becoming quieter and less communicative. He's been having dreams about his parents often, and he's becoming more and more unpredictable in his spontaneous decisions to stand.

Joe's daily routine now starts with an administrative assistant nurse from hospice giving Joe a bath with my assistance and then the nurse dressing him. For the first couple of weeks in December, Joe uses his walker with assistance and can go to the TV/breakfast area. He usually sits in his lift chair after he eats breakfast. He isn't doing much reading, though he occasionally goes online on his tablet. In the morning, Greg or I will usually spend time talking to him, or he naps, watches TV, or listens to classical music. He hasn't lost his appetite, and he continues to eat well. He loves ice cream—his current favorites are Häagen-Dazs vanilla Swiss almond and sea salt caramel gelato. Joe jokes about the Häagen-Dazs coming from Brooklyn even though the name sounds like it's from Germany or the Netherlands. He enjoys the marketing strategy a good name brings to his favorite ice cream.

We take Joe to the golf Learning Center at his request, as he wants to be around the sport he has played for so many years. He so wants to practice, but his balance and leg strength prevent him from doing so. Instead, we walk inside the facility and he looks around the golf shop. He makes eye contact with one of the working pros and they talk for a few minutes about golf clubs and the pro tour.

Joe is using his walker in the pro shop, and maneuvering through the racks of merchandise is a bit tricky, so I follow him to be there to help if he needs me. Then we go outside and he sits on a bench and watches golfers practice. He doesn't say much, and I assume he misses playing. Since we moved to Florida, we tried to play the six holes set up as practice for a short game twice. Both times Joe could use a putter, but not any clubs that required a backswing. He loves being outdoors and wants to try to play a little bit now, but it was frustrating for him because he felt unbalanced when he tried. We stay at the learning center for close to an hour before we leave.

Greg and Joe have many good conversations about learning to be successful working, relationships with friends and girlfriends, and generally just living and becoming more responsible. Joe is passing on to Greg whatever he thinks may help Greg after he's gone. He takes the opportunity several times to tell Greg how much he loves him and how proud he is of him. Greg also shares with his father how much he loves and respects him and how much he values the advice he's given him over the years and continues to give him now.

There's absolutely nothing about what's happening to Joe that I'm thankful about, but I do recognize that he and Greg are making the most of this time to be with each other and share so many thoughts and feelings. If we were to lose Joe suddenly—in a car accident, for example—they wouldn't have this opportunity.

◆

When the hospice nurse comes to see Joe, she checks his vital signs and records them in a notebook. I explain Joe's progression, especially how he's insisting more and more on standing up from his lift chair as if on impulse. Joe never regained his perception of time after his initial surgery, and now he has very little sense of intervals lengths. Occasionally Joe tells me he has a headache, and I'm allowed to give him ibuprofen or another NSAID* for the pain. It seems to help, though it makes him go to sleep. Joe continues to take his medicines for blood pressure, cholesterol, and IBD. As part of his initial evaluation, Joe was provided a bed with railings; eventually he's also given a portable toilet, bed pads, a respirator, and some other helpful personal hygiene items.

Greg and I have difficulty managing Joe's impulse to announce that he wants to stand. I explain it to the nurse each time she visits, and I ask what we should do. We aren't given a useful solution other than what we've already been doing, so it continues to happen with more and more frequency. Sometimes Joe tries to stand alone after he announces that he wants to stand, and other times he doesn't. Greg and I talk with Joe about it, and he agrees to give us some notice so we can help, but at least half the time he doesn't.

The third week of December, Greg's friend Colin stays with us for ten days during his break from pharmacy school. He's helped us with so many things during Joe's illness, and now he's helping again. Both Greg and Colin work out regularly and are very strong. Joe needs more physical assistance than I can provide alone, so having both Colin and Greg in the house is what Joe needs. Colin is so close to our family that we joked over the years that he's like Greg's part-time brother. It's a relief to me to have both the muscle help Greg and Colin provide, as well as the emotional support. All of us treat Joe as if he isn't sick: we engage him in conversation and involve him in decisions about what he wants to do during the day (however limited the options may be), his food choices, and friends that visit. Joe continues to have a few visitors, but not as many as before. He tires easily, and except for Bennett, most visitors are family.

Greg has always loved Christmas, the holiday spirit, decorations, and music. "Bah humbug!" Joe exclaims jokingly each year as we talk about decorating a tree for the holiday. Joe has long enjoyed pretending to be Scrooge around Christmas, although he really likes the holiday. This year I feel it's especially important to have a decorated Christmas tree, stockings, and a festive (although small) dinner. I find our Christmas CDs, including Kenny G, Barbara Streisand, Wilson Phillips, intermingled with Joe's favorite classical selections to listen to.

Try as I do to create a festive environment, I can't rid myself of the overriding desperation in my actions. Greg, Colin, and I put ornaments on the tree and playfully bicker about the best place to put them. Joe watches from his lift chair and laughs at our antics. Our two cats join in and nestle into the tree branches, taking playful swats at our hands as we add ornaments to the tree. My parents and Karen will be spending Christmas Day with us, and I'm so happy we'll be together.

◆

It's Wednesday, December 21—the winter solstice—and we're congratulating ourselves on being in Florida enjoying a mild sunny day. We checked the temperatures in Connecticut and noted they were in the low 30s, while here we are enjoying temperatures in the high 70s. I'm in the kitchen slicing a tomato for Joe's sandwich for lunch when I hear Joe announce he wants to stand. I put the knife down as he starts to stand, and in the time it takes me to walk the four strides to his chair, he stands, sways, and falls to his left. His legs are rigid, so it's as if he topples in a straight line. I rush forward and try to get under him, yelling, "No, no, no, don't fall!" But I'm not fast enough: Joe lands on his left shoulder and side, and his head hits the floor as well. I yell for Greg and Colin to join me, and the three of us quickly have Joe back in his seat. But already, a lump is forming on his forehead. Colin puts a cold compress on it to help reduce swelling, alternating 20 minutes on and 20 minutes off.

I call hospice as fast as I can and ask that a nurse come to our house immediately. I explain what happened, and they ask me about Joe's symptoms: they appear to be unchanged except for the bump. I know that any fall can be a problem, and I'm concerned that Joe hurt his shoulder or his side in the fall. But he can move his shoulder and arm and can twist without pain, which indicates no serious injury to the muscle or bone. I'm beside myself with worry that bumping his head will cause further damage, and I demand that a nurse come to our house immediately. The managing nurse tells me repeatedly to calm down, but I can't—especially when she says it will be 45 minutes before someone arrives. I ask if we should take him to the emergency room, but she says she'll send our nurse to our house next.

When our nurse arrives, she checks Joe's responsiveness and says he seems unchanged since she saw him last, noting that all his vital signs are normal. I ask that she call a hospice doctor to discuss his condition and I tell her I want to be on the call with her. The doctor tells us that if Joe experienced any additional brain issues from the fall, there would most likely be symptoms. The biggest concern would be any internal bleeding, and he describes what we should watch for: seizure, stroke, excessive sleeping, or other abnormalities that aren't in line with his current status. It's now been two hours since his fall, and nothing has changed. He's a very calming doctor to talk to, and we decide we'll watch Joe for any change in symptoms. Thank God there are none, although the bump on his forehead is unnerving.

I keep reliving in my mind what happened and I wonder if I could've done anything different or faster to stop it. I feel so guilty, like I didn't protect Joe, even though I don't know how I could've gotten to him any faster. I talk to the doctor about how Joe has been increasingly wanting to stand and how we never know when it'll happen. I explain that I've been asking hospice service about it for a couple of weeks, and I ask him if there's anything we can do about it. He says he thinks there's a medicine that can help, and he prescribes the same medicine Joe took to calm him when he had an MRI.

On Thursday, the hospice administrator calls to check on Joe, and I describe his symptoms. There are no changes other than that the muscles in his side are stiff from the fall, and his behavior is unchanged. She explains that they're assigning a new nurse to Joe, one with a great deal of experience with patients who have brain tumors. She'll be at our house later in the morning to evaluate Joe. I'm so happy about the news, and I welcome specialty care for Joe.

Joe's new nurse, Nurse P, arrives as scheduled, and we immediately observe a change in the level of care. She spends 30 minutes evaluating Joe's condition. After talking with the hospice physician, she administers the anti-anxiety medicine, explaining the dosage and interval. The nurse assistant who bathes Joe is also at our home, and the two of them spend some time discussing Joe's condition before Nurse P sits down to talk to me.

Nurse P is very easy to talk to. She's petite, wears light pink scrubs, and smiles a lot in a compassionate way. We're in the living room—Nurse P sitting on one striped sofa, me on the adjacent matching one. She explains that she's reviewed Joe's history and the case notes and then gathered her own information this morning. She discusses her background and nursing experience, which is mostly with brain-related illnesses. She pauses and asks me what I'd like to know about her assessment. I'm straightforward in my answer.

"I'd like to know everything you've found," I tell her. "Please don't hold anything back—I'd rather know than be 'protected' with limited information."

She nods and then proceeds to tell me what I asked for.

Nurse P tells me Joe is in a very advanced state of decline. The fact that I'm now feeding him (because of his severe essential tremor), his increased impulse to stand, decline in walking capability, balance issues, and his excessive sleeping (which indicates reduced engagement with us) are symptoms of this. She says she believes he has perhaps two or maybe three weeks. Joe's comfort is the most important thing at this point, and she assures me that the hospice staff will help. She also helps me understand what to expect: she believes that Joe will begin to have headaches and hallucinations, will eventually stop talking and eating, and will appear to be in a coma. She believes Joe will understand what is happening around him and will be able to hear but won't be able to respond.

Well, I wanted to have the straight direct facts, and I have them now. I imagine this is what it feels like to be hit by a Mack truck. Being with Joe day after day, I'm not noticing the decline easily. And of course, there's the fact that I can't really accept that he isn't going to be with me—and soon. I've been told but have been unable to believe or accept it. My friends' panic, desperation, fear and anger are circling me like buzzards waiting for a feeding frenzy.

◆

It's Christmas 2016—another crisp, 80-degree day with sunshine that brings light into the house as we spend a family day together. Everyone but me is sleeping later than usual, and I'm the first one up and about. I prepare a light Christmas breakfast, knowing we'll be having a big meal later. I take food into our room to see if Joe would like to eat. He's still quietly sleeping, so I don't wake him up to eat. It can be reheated when he's ready.

Gradually everyone else wakes up—first Greg, then Colin, and then my parents. But Joe is still asleep. We hold off on opening presents and enjoy Christmas music and family time. Both Simba and Rascal know something is up, so they prowl around the Christmas tree, then move from one lap to another. We eat our light breakfast and then watch "Miracle on 34th Street" for the 100th time. My mom and I stuff the small turkey we have and prepare sweet potato casserole, green beans, and salad for our Christmas dinner.

I decide to wake Joe up, so I talk to him while I raise the back of his automated bed. He wakes up groggy. "Merry Christmas, sleepyhead!" I exclaim. I ask him if he wants go to the TV room and open presents, but he shakes his head no.

"Then we'll bring your presents here and celebrate with you!" I tell him.

He nods yes and points to his cup. I ask him if he wants orange juice, and he nods yes. I bring him some and help him put the straw to his mouth so he can drink. Greg and Colin bring his presents into the room and place them on the bed next to his. My parents and Karen join us also. Joe puts his juice down and reaches for a present. Greg hands it to him, but as he tries to open it, the present drops to the floor. His hands are shaking so very much. I pick the present up and offer to help him open it. He nods yes. Each gift is opened that way, and Joe motions for me to write down what each gift is and who gave it to him. He still always wants to be sure to thank anyone who gives him a present, and every year at Christmas, he makes a list of gifts and givers. This year he gets a University of Tennessee blanket, hat, and beer cup, plus some books, pullover shirts, and music. He smiles as each gift is opened and nods his thanks. He tries to talk, but his voice is so very quiet and raspy. We're surrounding him, trying to bring him a little cheer.

After the presents are opened, he leans back into his pillows. I ask him if he'd like some food, and he nods yes. After the crowd leaves the room, Greg and I stay with him while I feed him his late breakfast. I chatter about Christmas and try to convince Joe to come into the TV room, but he shakes his head no and says he's tired. I clear his breakfast plate and go back to his room. Then I sit on our bed, which is pushed up next to the hospital bed Joe is resting in. I stay with him, holding on to his right arm while he sleeps.

◆

Joe, Greg, and I have never missed a Christmas together. We haven't always spent Christmas Day at our house—sometimes we were at Joe's parents' house, my parents', or the home of one of my sisters. Our Christmas Days, wherever we were, always have the same rituals. Usually we attend Mass the evening before, but occasionally we attend Mass on Christmas morning. When Greg was younger, we'd go to Mass the afternoon before so we could open presents first thing in the morning. Afterward, Greg and Joe would spend time together playing video games or some other activity while I would prepare our Christmas meal. The house would be filled with the smell of turkey, and we'd be hungry for a mid-afternoon meal.

If we were visiting relatives, the men would often leave for a few hours to try to find a golf course that was open so they could play. Greg would stay and spend time with his cousins, or he'd go play golf with Joe if his cousins weren't with us. We've always spent Christmas with family for the entire day. I want to be with Joe the entire day today also. But today he seems content to sleep and stay in his hospital bed. That has never happened since he became ill, and I stay with him most of the day, leaving him only to help with the cooking and preparations for dinner.

I bring a plate of Christmas dinner to Joe to eat mid-afternoon. I feed him slowly, and he eats a decent portion of food. He loves turkey, stuffing, and gravy, and he seems to enjoy his food. When he's finished, I read to him from one of his new books. He closes his eyes and appears to be listening, but then I realize he's breathing deeply and is asleep. Greg joins me, and we stare at each other across Joe sleeping in his bed. As hard as I try to control myself, I can't, and tears are sliding down my cheeks before I can stop them. Greg is also teary eyed as we both try to come to terms with what's happening.

My parents leave the day after Christmas, and Peggy comes to stay with us. I called hospice on Tuesday morning to let them know Joe isn't getting out of bed anymore. They continue to provide care for Joe, giving him bed baths and instructing me on how to care for Joe's hygiene when they're not at our home. I contact Joe's siblings and friend Bennett to let them know Joe's end is near.

◆

Christmas Day was the last time Joe ate or drank anything. His eyes aren't open often, and when they are, he's staring to his right at the ceiling. The hospice nurses tell me he can hear what's being said to him, and they encourage me and Greg to talk to him, which we do constantly throughout the day when his eyes are open. I read to him and read a prayer to him every day. I call our new parish and ask for a priest to come to our home and administer last rites to Joe. My parents, my sisters, Joe's siblings, and Bennett come to see Joe for a final visit. They talk to Joe, and I believe he hears what is said to him.

Hospice nurses are with Joe 24/7 now and set up a nurse's table in our bedroom. Each nurse stays one night and then usually returns for a second night. Every couple of days or so, a different nurse comes to our home. They're all very qualified, caring, and compassionate toward Joe and our family. They administer Joe's medicine through an IV* as he's not swallowing anymore. Each day I continue to pray for

Joe to be saved, however futile I know it is. The pain is unbearable, watching Joe lie in his bed day after day, not seeming to know us anymore. I talk to him, update him on current affairs, read to him, tell him how much I love him—anything I can think of to be near him, even if he really can't hear me. Who really knows? But as long as he's still here, I can cope.

My anger at the cruel state of affairs continues to build. I do pray, but I don't understand why we have been let down. How could God let Joe have this illness and suffer through so much this year? Each nurse who comes to our home, I try to welcome as much as I can. I'm not thinking very clearly at this point, but I do try to learn a little about them. Because after all, what a help they are to us, and isn't that what Joe would do if he could speak? It's beyond my comprehension that they can actually come to someone's home and help in the ways they do. God bless the nurses of this world.

One night when I'm feeling especially angry at God, our hospice nurse, Nurse N, starts telling me a little about her family. Her father is a minister who was diagnosed with lung cancer, had treatment, and was in remission. As a minister, he would talk to his parish about his illness and praise God for helping him. Recently he was told that his cancer had returned. He found his feelings had changed and he started to feel bitter, starting to feel anger over his situation. I can completely relate to her story. He began wondering why God was letting him go through this *a second time*. Then, as if a light came on, he realized that God did not create the illnesses we succumb to. WE create these illnesses, from our lifestyle. Whether it be from smoking, what we eat or drink, byproducts of chemical processes—who knows? God helps us cope with what we're dealing with, but is not the origin of it.

Now, I hadn't spoken of my feelings on this subject to anyone. Was it simply a coincidence that Nurse N told me the story? I think not, and it really helped me stop fueling my anger. It also reminded me of all the help Joe and I had over his yearlong illness and recognize that we were getting help with coping with Joe's illness. What is the phrase —"gratitude or desire"? Even in the direst of circumstances, I find reason to be grateful for the help we have.

Day in and day out, for eighteen days straight, Joe doesn't eat or drink. The hospice nurses express surprise that Joe is holding on as long as he is. They tell Greg and me that it's as if Joe needs some reassurance from us so he can leave us. We're advised to assure Joe that we'll be okay if he leaves. So even though I don't believe it, I tell him. I also tell him over and over how much I love him and will miss him. I talk to him about his parents, how he'll be reunited with them, his cousin Jim, and his friend Brian. Greg also tells Joe how he loves him and will miss him but that he'll be okay. I really don't know if Joe can hear or understand us, but I don't want to be the cause of him lingering in his condition. The priest from our new parish comes to our home and administers last rites to Joe. Bennett visits with his family and has a few last moments with him—his chance to talk to Joe a final time.

Greg and I don't know what's going on in Joe's mind at this point. The contrast between the life he's led and his current state is pitiful. Such intelligence, now in a coma-like state. We don't know what to expect next, and we're standing by to do anything the nurse needs help with. Joe is administered morphine for his pain as needed. I rest on the couch next to the open bedroom door each night, ready to help as needed.

At 3 a.m. on January 13—exactly one year from the day Joe was diagnosed with his illness—the nurse calls for me. She tells me she thinks it's Joe's time to leave. I call for Greg, and he quickly joins us. Simba and Rascal are pressed against Joe's sides. We're with Joe for his last moments on earth, praying over him—our small family united together for the last time.

Epilogue

Memories can be a tricky thing. After all, who's to say they aren't accurate when only you are recollecting? That's how I feel about the days following Joe's passing. I remember being with Joe when he passed, and I remember the funeral home staff collecting Joe's body. I remember notifying Joe's brother and sister and my family. I remember my sister Peggy coming to our home and helping Greg and me sort through Joe's belongings. I recall coordinating with Bennett, who was so very helpful with notifying many of Joe's friends and colleagues of his passing. I remember driving with Greg to my hometown for Joe's funeral. There must be many things I don't remember, as there are gaps in the days after Joe's passing. I knew better than to drink any alcohol, as I'm sure it would have led to further memory gaps and unrestrained grief.

The trip to the funeral is blurry. I remember it didn't rain and the roads weren't very busy. Greg and I stayed at my parents' house the night before the funeral service. Preparations for Joe's funeral had been made in advance, although we didn't know the timing. The service was held at Resurrection Catholic Church at 10:30 a.m. on January 21, 2017, followed by a memorial luncheon at Grassland Country Club and interment at Oak Hill Cemetery. Gentry-Morrison Funeral Home handled all the arrangements, including Joe's remains, sign-in book, coordination with the church and cemetery, memorial website, video, and flowers. I selected readings, music, and speakers for the service and memorial luncheon, as well as the menu. My sisters handled anything else that came up during the service, luncheon, and interment. I was in no condition to do anything other than try to talk to those who wished to pay last respects to Joe and express their condolences to me and Greg and our families. I remember that many people attended Joe's funeral, and I believe I spoke to most of them, although I can't recall a word I said.

I do remember that I was impressed that Joe's family, including many of his cousins, traveled a long distance to attend the services and pay their respects. Many people went to a great deal of effort to travel from Connecticut and from other areas of Florida. Their attendance is a testament to Joe's character and to his strong bonds with his family, friends, and colleagues who supported him throughout his illness. There was an overwhelming feeling of loss, and so much love for Joe.

I thank each of you on behalf of Joe. I believe he shared this day with us, smiling down at us as we honored him at his service, memorial lunch, and interment. I like to think he would have enjoyed being with all of you one last time if he could have been with us in person. He would have been the last to leave the party.

Many of Joe's colleagues couldn't travel to his funeral. They arranged a dedication to Joe at his place of work in February 2017 and named a conference room in is honor. It was my privilege to attend this dedication. Being the humble person Joe was, I believe he would have been slightly embarrassed by the attention, but nonetheless pleased. Thanks to each of you who participated in this honor.

There are many of you who have traveled a similar journey with a loved one, whether a life partner, parent, sibling, or friend. There's no solace for what we have lost, no defined path for our future. We stumble through each day looking for what is no longer available to us. We learn to cope and to get through each day, but never do we forget or find a substitute—there is none.

Joe died of an incurable disease, but it is constantly being researched. Net proceeds from the sale of this book will be donated to Massachusetts General Hospital and Treasure Coast Hospice to support their efforts to find a cure—or in the meantime, to at least preserve the dignity and quality of life of those we love as they battle this devastating disease. We know we can't live forever, but perhaps we can have more quality time with those we love.

APPENDIX

Part A. Chapter Notes

These notes expand on and clarify content within the book indicated by an asterisk (*). After each note is the URL of the website where the information is available. Check out those websites for more useful information.

Chapter 1

MRI: a procedure in which radio waves and a powerful magnet linked to a computer are used to create pictures of areas in the body. These pictures can show the difference between normal and diseased tissue. MRI makes better images of organs and soft tissue than other scanning techniques, such as computed tomography (CT) or x-ray. MRI is especially useful for imaging the brain, the spine, the soft tissue of joints, and the inside of bones. Also called magnetic resonance imaging. https://www.cancer.gov/publications/dictionaries/cancer-terms/def/mri

Brain anomaly: a brain anomaly, or brain abnormality, is any feature of the brain that is not typical. Some are present at birth. Others develop over time. A brain abnormality can indicate any of several problems, like Down syndrome, dementia, or a tumor. https://link.springer.com/referenceworkentry/10.1007%2F978-0-387-79061-9_406

Neurology specialist (neurologist): a doctor who has special training in diagnosing and treating disorders of the nervous system. https://

www.cancer.gov/publications/dictionaries/cancer-terms/def/neurologist

Brain tumor: an abnormal mass of tissue that results when cells divide more than they should or do not die when they should. A brain tumor is a tumor in the tissues of the brain. Tumors can be benign (not cancer) or malignant (cancer). https://www.cancer.gov/publications/dictionaries/cancer-terms/def/brain-tumor https://www.cancer.gov/publications/dictionaries/cancer-terms/def/tumor

Biopsy: the removal of cells or tissues from the body for examination or testing. A doctor may examine the cells or tissues under a microscope or perform other tests on them. The purpose of a biopsy is to try to see if there is a disease in the cells or tissues and, if so, get information about the disease. https://www.cancer.gov/publications/dictionaries/cancer-terms/def/tumor

Glioma: a type of brain cancer that begins in glial cells (cells that surround and support nerve cells). https://www.cancer.gov/publications/dictionaries/cancer-terms/def/glioma

Chemotherapy: treatment that uses drugs to stop the growth of cancer cells, either by killing the cells or by stopping them from dividing. It is sometimes given with other types of treatments. https://www.cancer.gov/publications/dictionaries/cancer-terms/def/chemotherapy

Radiation therapy: the use of high-energy radiation from x-rays, gamma rays, neutrons, protons, and other sources to kill cancer cells and shrink tumors. https://www.cancer.gov/publications/dictionaries/cancer-terms/def/44971

Resection: surgery to remove tissue or part or all of an organ. https://www.cancer.gov/publications/dictionaries/cancer-terms/def/resection

Steroid drug: a type of drug used to relieve swelling and inflammation. Some steroid drugs may also treat tumors. https://www.cancer.gov/publications/dictionaries/cancer-terms/def/steroid-drug

Neurosurgeon: a doctor who has special training in surgery on the brain, spine, and other parts of the nervous system. https://www.cancer.gov/publications/dictionaries/cancer-terms/def/neurosurgeon

Glioblastoma: a fast-growing type of tumor that forms from glial (supportive) tissue of the brain and spinal cord. Also called glioblastoma multiforme, GBM, and grade IV astrocytoma. https://www.cancer.gov/publications/dictionaries/cancer-terms/def/glioblastoma

Wikipedia: Wikipedia is a very popular website for finding general information. But even the site itself warns to be cautious about its reliability, noting:

We advise special caution when using Wikipedia as a source for research. Anyone may edit an article, deleting accurate information or adding false information.

However, Wikipedia can be a useful starting point by looking at the reference list within each article, which might include reputable sources of information.

Crohn's disease: a condition in which the gastrointestinal tract (part of the digestive system) is inflamed over a long period of time. Crohn's disease usually affects the small intestine and colon. https://www.cancer.gov/publications/dictionaries/cancer-terms/def/crohn-disease

Chapter 2

Vital signs: measurements that show how well your body is functioning. They include **blood pressure, heart rate, respiratory rate (breathing), and body temperature.** https://medlineplus.gov/vitalsigns.html

Anesthesiologist: a doctor who has special training in giving drugs or other agents to prevent or relieve pain during surgery or other medical procedures. https://www.cancer.gov/publications/dictionaries/cancer-terms/def/anesthesiologist

Propofol: a drug commonly used for general anesthesia to make a person sleepy during surgery or some other medical procedure. https://www.rxlist.com/consumer_propofol_diprivan/drugs-condition.htm

Craniotomy: an operation in which a piece of the skull is removed. A craniotomy may be done to remove abnormal brain tissue. https://www.cancer.gov/publications/dictionaries/cancer-terms/def/craniotomy

Pathology report: the description of cells and tissues based on what is examined under a microscope. A pathology report is sometimes used to make a diagnosis of a disease. https://www.cancer.gov/publications/dictionaries/cancer-terms/def/pathology-report

Catheter: a flexible tube used to deliver fluids into the body or withdraw fluids from the body. https://www.cancer.gov/publications/dictionaries/cancer-terms/def/catheter

Physical therapist: a health professional trained to evaluate people who have conditions or injuries that limit their ability to do physical activities. After evaluating a patient, the physical therapist treats the patient by using exercises and other methods to help improve movement. https://www.cancer.gov/publications/dictionaries/cancer-terms/def/physical-therapist

Occupational therapist: a health professional trained to help people learn to manage their daily activities. https://www.cancer.gov/publications/dictionaries/cancer-terms/def/occupational-therapist

Radiation oncologist: a doctor who has special training in using radiation to treat cancer. https://www.cancer.gov/publications/dictionaries/cancer-terms/def/radiation-oncologist

Neuro-oncologist: a doctor who has special training in diagnosing and treating brain tumors and other tumors of the nervous system. https://www.cancer.gov/publications/dictionaries/cancer-terms/def/neuro-oncologist

Chapter 3

Incentive spirometer: a device that helps people breathe more deeply and more comfortably after surgery. https://medlineplus.gov/ency/patientinstructions/000451.htm

FDA regulation of dietary supplements: *The U.S. Food and Drug Administration (FDA) does not have the authority to review dietary supplement products for safety and effectiveness before they are marketed. That means supplements can be sold before they're proven effective, and they may have health risks. The FDA website has information about supplements at:* https://www.fda.gov/food/dietary-supplements/information-consumers-using-dietary-supplements

Symptoms of lesions in the frontal lobes: There are four lobes in each of the two sides of your brain; each lobe has a different function, which will be affected depending on the location of the lesion or damage:

- Frontal lobe: cognitive functions, voluntary movement
- Parietal lobe: temperature, taste, touch, and movement
- Occipital lobe: vision
- Temporal lobe: links the sensations of taste, sound, sight, and touch to memories

https://www.mayoclinic.org/brain-lobes/img-20008887

Cumulative effects: with each radiation treatment, the effects are more pronounced than those produced by the first treatment. https://www.medilexicon.com/dictionary/28009

CT scan (computed tomography scan) or CAT scan (computed axial tomography scan): a procedure that uses a computer linked to an x-ray machine to take pictures of areas in the body. A CT scan may be used to help diagnose disease, plan treatment, or find out how well treatment is working. https://www.cancer.gov/publications/dictionaries/cancer-terms/def/ct-scan

Bevacizumab + lomustine; bevacizumab + temozolomide: two types of combination therapies (two or more drugs used together). These therapies treat some types of gliomas, but the success rate is very low for glioblastoma multiforme, unmethylated, grade IV astrocytoma. At the time, they were among the best options available. Weller M, Cloughesy T, Perry JR, Wick W. Standards of care for treatment of recurrent glioblastoma--are we there yet? *Neuro Oncol.* 2013;15(1):4–27. doi:10.1093/neuonc/nos273

Clinical trials: This is a useful resource for general information about what clinical trials are and what trials are currently available: https://clinicaltrials.gov/

EGFR (epidermal growth factor receptor): a protein found at abnormally high levels on the surface of many types of cancer cells. https://www.cancer.gov/publications/dictionaries/cancer-terms/def/egfr

Phase 2 clinical trial: a phase is the stage of a study, based on factors like the goal of the study and the number of people participating in it. There are five phases: early phase 1 (formerly listed as phase 0), phase 1, phase 2, phase 3, and phase 4. https://clinicaltrials.gov/ct2/about-studies/glossary

Immunotherapy: the immune system is a network of cells, tissues, organs, and the substances that they make. All of these work together to help fight cancer, infection, and other diseases. Immunotherapy stimulates or suppresses the immune system to help the body fight disease. https://www.cancer.gov/publications/dictionaries/cancer-terms/def/immunotherapy

https://www.cancer.gov/publications/dictionaries/cancer-terms/def/immune-system

Clinical trials: These are useful resources for details about clinical trials:

- https://www.clinicaltrials.gov/ct2/help/glossary/phase
- https://www.cancer.org/treatment/treatments-and-side-effects/clinical-trials/what-you-need-to-know/phases-of-clinical-trials.html

Chapter 4

Infusion: another name for IV (intravenous infusion)—a way of putting drugs or other fluids into the bloodstream. https://www.cancer.gov/publications/dictionaries/cancer-terms/def/infusion

Cumulative effects: with each radiation treatment, the effects are more pronounced than those produced by the first treatment. https://www.medilexicon.com/dictionary/28009

3-dimensional conformal radiation therapy: a procedure that uses a computer to create a 3-dimensional picture of the tumor. This allows doctors to give the highest possible dose of radiation to the tumor while limiting the effect on the normal tissue. Also called 3-dimensional radiation therapy and 3D-CRT. https://www.cancer.gov/publications/dictionaries/cancer-terms/def/3-dimensional-conformal-radiation-therapy

"Don't believe everything you read on the Internet": When you're looking for health information, it can be challenging to find reliable sources. This is especially true with online resources, because anyone can write whatever they want and make it look authentic. These resources can help you figure out whether the information is timely, verified, and accurate.

- https://medlineplus.gov/evaluatinghealthinformation.html
- https://www.genome.gov/Genetic-and-Rare-Diseases-Information-Center/Finding-reliable-health-information
- https://www.jointcommission.org/patient_101_how_to_find_reliable_health_information/

Adverse reaction: a harmful and unintended response to a medicine or treatment. http://apps.who.int/medicinedocs/en/d/Jh2992e/2.html

Essential tremor: a type of involuntary shaking movement. It has no known cause. https://medlineplus.gov/ency/article/000762.htm

Chapter 5

Functions of the frontal lobe: the frontal lobe is important to these functions, so people with damage to the frontal lobe may have trouble with tasks related to them:

- Gathering information
- Remembering previous experiences
- Decision making
- Speech
- Some voluntary movements
- **Making comparisons**
- Empathy
- Personality
- Motivation
- Paying attention

https://www.medicalnewstoday.com/articles/318139.php

Comprehensive metabolic panel: a group of blood tests that indicate the body's chemical balance and metabolism. Metabolism refers to how the body uses energy. https://medlineplus.gov/ency/article/003468.htm

LDH: a substance in body tissues that is involved in energy production in cells. An increased amount in the blood may be a sign of tissue damage and some types of cancer or other diseases. https://www.cancer.gov/publications/dictionaries/cancer-terms/def/ldh

CBC with differential: a measure of the number of different types of cells in the blood. It is used to help diagnose and monitor various health conditions. https://www.cancer.gov/publications/dictionaries/cancer-terms/def/cbc-with-differential

IV: into or within a vein. IV usually refers to a way of giving a drug or other substance through a needle or tube inserted into a vein. Also called intravenous. https://www.cancer.gov/publications/dictionaries/cancer-terms/def/iv

Clinical trials: This is a useful resource for general information about what clinical trials are and what trials are currently available: https://clinicaltrials.gov/

Patient portal: a secure online website that gives patients convenient, 24-hour access to personal health information from anywhere with an Internet connection. Each person uses a different secure username and password to view their health information. Some patient portals also allow you to communicate with your doctor, schedule appointments, and view educational materials. https://www.healthit.gov/faq/what-patient-portal

Crohn's disease: a condition in which the gastrointestinal tract (part of the digestive system) is inflamed over a long period of time. Crohn's disease usually affects the small intestine and colon. https://www.cancer.gov/publications/dictionaries/cancer-terms/def/crohn-disease

T2-hyperintensity: T2 refers to the type of contrast used in the MRI. Hyperintensity refers to the concentration of darkness on the MRI. It may indicate growth of cancer cells in this case. https://

casemed.case.edu/clerkships/neurology/Web%20Neurorad/MRI%20Basics.htm

Dexamethasone: a corticosteroid drug used to reduce inflammation (swelling) and lower the body's immune response. It is used with other drugs to treat some types of cancer. It is also used to treat or prevent some conditions related to cancer and cancer treatment. https://www.cancer.gov/publications/dictionaries/cancer-terms/def/dexamethasone/steroid

Bevacizumab + lomustine; bevacizumab + temozolomide: two types of combination therapies (two or more drugs used together). These therapies treat some types of gliomas, but the success rate is very low for glioblastoma multiforme, unmethylated, grade IV astrocytoma. At the time, they were among the best options available. Weller M, Cloughesy T, Perry JR, Wick W. Standards of care for treatment of recurrent glioblastoma--are we there yet? *Neuro Oncol.* 2013;15(1):4–27. doi:10.1093/neuonc/nos273

Tumor progression: change in the traits of a tumor that indicate the growth of abnormal cells. https://www.sciencedirect.com/topics/medicine-and-dentistry/tumor-progression

"…on the Internet, it says some people live three to five years." In reality, most people with GBM live an average of fifteen to sixteen months. It's very rare for someone to live more than five years, although new research seems to be improving those numbers slowly. https://www.healthline.com/health/brain-tumor/glioblastoma#survival-rates-and-life-expectancy

Common end-of-life symptoms for people with brain cancer include severe fatigue and weakness, problems eating, problems with digestion and bodily functions, vomiting, difficulty swallowing, breathing problems, confusion, agitation, and depression. Each person's symptoms may vary greatly depending on the size, location, and progression of the tumor. https://www.ucsfhealth.org/pdf/transition_of_care_handbook.pdf

Chapter 6

Fentanyl: a drug used to treat severe pain from cancer when opioids are not effective enough. It is also used during anesthesia for surgery. https://www.cancer.gov/publications/dictionaries/cancer-terms/def/fentanyl-citrate

G-tube (gastrostomy tube): a tube inserted directly into the stomach. It can be used to give a patient drugs and liquids, including liquid food. It also allows air and fluid to leave the stomach. https://www.cancer.gov/publications/dictionaries/cancer-terms/def/gastrostomy-tube

PICC line (peripherally inserted central catheter): a medical device used to draw blood and give treatments, including IV fluids, drugs, or blood transfusions. A thin, flexible tube is inserted, running from a vein in the arm to a vein in the heart. It may stay in place for weeks or months, so it helps avoid the need for repeated needle sticks. https://www.cancer.gov/publications/dictionaries/cancer-terms/def/picc

Laparoscopically: performed using a laparoscope—a thin, tube-like instrument used to look at tissues and organs inside the abdomen. A laparoscope may have a tool to remove tissue. https://www.cancer.gov/publications/dictionaries/cancer-terms/def/laparoscope

Oxygen percentage: the level of oxygen in your blood. A normal oxygen percentage is about 95 percent to 100 percent. A low oxygen percentage may be a sign of a problem with breathing or circulation.

https://www.mayoclinic.org/symptoms/hypoxemia/basics/definition/sym-20050930

Remission: a decrease in signs and symptoms of cancer (partial remission) or a disappearance of signs and symptoms of cancer (complete remission). https://www.cancer.gov/publications/dictionaries/cancer-terms/def/remission

Chapter 7

MRI, with or without contrast: an MRI is a procedure in which radio waves and a powerful magnet linked to a computer are used to create pictures of areas in the body. Most MRIs do not require contrast. For some MRIs, the doctor may request a contrast (dye), which is given through an IV. The contrast helps the radiologist see some areas more clearly. https://medlineplus.gov/ency/article/003335.htm

The glioma may have spread through spinal fluid and elsewhere: most astrocytomas can spread widely throughout the brain. Sometimes they spread along the cerebrospinal fluid (CSF) pathways. It is very rare for them to spread outside of the brain or spinal cord. https://www.cancer.org/cancer/brain-spinal-cord-tumors-adults/about/types-of-brain-tumors.html

Cervical MRI scan: an MRI of the portion of your spine that runs through the neck area. https://medlineplus.gov/ency/article/007354.htm

Lumbar MRI scan: an MRI of the lower portion of the spine. https://medlineplus.gov/ency/article/007352.htm

EEG to identify seizure risk: an electroencephalogram (EEG) is a test to measure the electrical activity of the brain. Abnormal brain activity may indicate a seizure. https://medlineplus.gov/ency/article/003931.htm

Disease progression: the spreading or growth of cancer. https://www.cancer.gov/publications/dictionaries/cancer-terms/def/disease-progression

An anticonvulsant and an antacid: A side effect of the anticonvulsant medicine is problems with the stomach and digestion. An antacid medicine was prescribed to ease the side effects of the anticonvulsant. The antacid was not prescribed specifically for the cancer.

Hospice facility: There are different levels of care for long-term illnesses. With palliative care, a patient can continue regular treatment while the palliative treatment focuses on pain and other symptoms. Find more information here:

https://www.webmd.com/palliative-care/when-is-palliative-care-appropriate#1

"I mention that Joe is getting up two or three times a night and appears quite restless, almost as if it's a spontaneous reaction to something." This was confusing and worrisome at the time, but we soon learned that it was a sign of more damage to the frontal lobe and wasn't dangerous.

Hospice/end-of-life care: when a disease is incurable and treatment isn't working, hospice care focuses on quality of life instead of a cure. Find more information here:

https://www.webmd.com/healthy-aging/hospice-care#1

Chapter 8

Incidence: the number of new cases of a disease diagnosed each year. https://www.cancer.gov/publications/dictionaries/cancer-terms/def/incidence

Glioblastoma multiforme (GBM): ***glioblastoma:*** a fast-growing type of tumor that forms from glial (supportive) tissue of the brain and spinal cord. Also called glioblastoma multiforme, GBM, and grade IV astrocytoma. https://www.cancer.gov/publications/dictionaries/cancer-terms/def/glioblastoma

Primary brain tumor: a tumor that starts in the brain. Cancer cells from a primary tumor may spread to other parts of the body and form new tumors, called secondary tumors. This is called metastasis. https://www.cancer.gov/publications/dictionaries/cancer-terms/def/primary-tumor

Metastatic brain tumors: secondary brain tumors—brain tumors that spread from primary tumors in a different part of the body. https://www.cancer.gov/publications/dictionaries/cancer-terms/def/primary-tumor

Remission: a decrease or disappearance in signs and symptoms of cancer or other disease https://www.cancer.gov/publications/dictionaries/cancer-terms/def/remission

NSAIDs (non-steroidal anti-inflammatory drugs): drugs that treat pain, fever, and inflammation. C**ommon over-the-counter (OTC) NSAIDs are** ibuprofen and naproxen. https://www.arthritis-health.com/glossary/non-steroidal-anti-inflammatory-drugs-nsaids

IV: into or within a vein. IV usually refers to a way of giving a drug or other substance through a needle or tube inserted into a vein. Also called intravenous. https://www.cancer.gov/publications/dictionaries/cancer-terms/def/iv

Part B: Useful Resources

Knowledge is power. And knowing how to get that knowledge can help you be a health advocate for yourself or for someone you care about. These are some valuable sources of information that can help you do that. You can find more information in the references in the Chapter Notes sections.

Specific to brain cancer

The American Brain Tumor Association: www.abta.org

General cancer resources

National Cancer Society: www.cancer.gov

American Cancer Society: www.cancer.org

Support for caregivers

Family Caregiver Alliance: www.caregiver.org

Brain cancer research

www.cancer.gov/types/brain/research

Clinical trials

https://clinicaltrials.gov

Dictionary of terms related to cancer

www.cancer.gov/publicatons/dictionaries/cancer-terms

Massachusetts General Hospital Cancer Center

www.massgeneral.org/cancer

Cognitive rehabilitation—a method of restoring cognitive function after brain surgery, stroke, brain injury, or some other trauma to the brain.

https://itspsychology.com/cognitive-rehabilitation/

Searching Looking for Reliable Information

When you're looking for health information, it can be challenging to figure out whether a source is reliable. This is especially true with online resources, because anyone can write whatever they want and make it look professional. These resources can help you figure out whether the information is timely, verified, and accurate.

https://medlineplus.gov/evaluatinghealthinformation.html

https://www.genome.gov/Genetic-and-Rare-Diseases-Information-Center/Finding-reliable-health-information

https://www.jointcommission.org/patient_101_how_to_find_reliable_health_information/

Things I Learned

- Spend as much time as you can with those you love.
- Live your life along the way. Don't continue to save, thinking you'll have time at the end to enjoy it. None of us know what is in store for us.
- Have your affairs in order, including your life style plan, financials, will and estate planning, and funeral wishes.
- Have medical insurance.
- Know your insurance coverage.
- Always contact your insurance company before any test or procedure is completed—even if your doctor's office says it's approved. And get a letter from your insurance company with approval for each procedure.
- If you're employed, understand your company's disability coverage.
- Learn all you can about your diagnosis.
- Ask your doctor any questions you want to.
- Get a second opinion for any major medical diagnosis.
- Use all resources available to you.
- Accept help from others.
- Buy, rent, or borrow medical equipment recommended by physical and occupational therapists.
- A lift chair can be very helpful.
- Create a medicine spreadsheet.
- Eat balanced and nutritional food, as recommended by your doctor.

- Follow your medication schedule exactly.
- Prepare your home to accommodate the patient.
- Use a showerhead extension hose.
- Sleep when the patient sleeps.
- If you're a caregiver, remember to take care of yourself, too.
- Use a pillbox for organizing medicine.
- Have a wheelchair handy.

CPSIA information can be obtained
at www.ICGtesting.com
Printed in the USA
FFHW010901051119

9 780578 563121